Advancing Ge[barcode]~ted
Therapies f
Nervous Syste...

PROCEEDINGS OF A WORKSHOP

Lisa Bain and Clare Stroud, *Rapporteurs*

Forum on Neuroscience and Nervous System Disorders

Board on Health Sciences Policy

Health and Medicine Division

The National Academies of
SCIENCES · ENGINEERING · MEDICINE

THE NATIONAL ACADEMIES PRESS
Washington, DC
www.nap.edu

THE NATIONAL ACADEMIES PRESS   500 Fifth Street, NW   Washington, DC 20001

This activity was supported by contracts between the National Academy of Sciences and Alzheimer's Association; Cohen Veterans Bioscience; Department of Health and Human Services' Food and Drug Administration (5R13FD005362-02) and National Institutes of Health (NIH) (HHSN26300089 [Under Master Base #DHHS-10002880]) through the National Center for Complementary and Integrative Health, National Eye Institute, National Institute of Mental Health, National Institute of Neurological Disorders and Stroke, National Institute on Aging, National Institute on Alcohol Abuse and Alcoholism, National Institute on Drug Abuse, and NIH Blueprint for Neuroscience Research; Department of Veterans Affairs (VA240-14-C-0057); Eli Lilly and Company; Foundation for the National Institutes of Health; Gatsby Charitable Foundation; Janssen Research & Development, LLC; The Kavli Foundation; Lundbeck Research USA; Merck Research Laboratories; The Michael J. Fox Foundation for Parkinson's Research; National Multiple Sclerosis Society; National Science Foundation (BCS-1064270); One Mind; Sanofi; Society for Neuroscience; Takeda Pharmaceuticals International, Inc.; The University of Rhode Island; and Wellcome Trust. Any opinions, findings, conclusions, or recommendations expressed in this publication do not necessarily reflect the views of any organization or agency that provided support for the project.

International Standard Book Number-13: 978-0-309-49584-4
International Standard Book Number-10: 0-309-49584-9
Digital Object Identifier: https://doi.org/10.17226/25529

Additional copies of this publication are available from the National Academies Press, 500 Fifth Street, NW, Keck 360, Washington, DC 20001; (800) 624-6242 or (202) 334-3313; http://www.nap.edu.

Printed in the United States of America

Suggested citation: National Academies of Sciences, Engineering, and Medicine. 2019. *Advancing gene-targeted therapies for central nervous system disorders: Proceedings of a workshop*. Washington, DC: The National Academies Press. https://doi.org/10.17226/25529.

The National Academies of
SCIENCES · ENGINEERING · MEDICINE

The **National Academy of Sciences** was established in 1863 by an Act of Congress, signed by President Lincoln, as a private, nongovernmental institution to advise the nation on issues related to science and technology. Members are elected by their peers for outstanding contributions to research. Dr. Marcia McNutt is president.

The **National Academy of Engineering** was established in 1964 under the charter of the National Academy of Sciences to bring the practices of engineering to advising the nation. Members are elected by their peers for extraordinary contributions to engineering. Dr. John L. Anderson is president.

The **National Academy of Medicine** (formerly the Institute of Medicine) was established in 1970 under the charter of the National Academy of Sciences to advise the nation on medical and health issues. Members are elected by their peers for distinguished contributions to medicine and health. Dr. Victor J. Dzau is president.

The three Academies work together as the **National Academies of Sciences, Engineering, and Medicine** to provide independent, objective analysis and advice to the nation and conduct other activities to solve complex problems and inform public policy decisions. The National Academies also encourage education and research, recognize outstanding contributions to knowledge, and increase public understanding in matters of science, engineering, and medicine.

Learn more about the National Academies of Sciences, Engineering, and Medicine at **www.nationalacademies.org**.

The National Academies of
SCIENCES · ENGINEERING · MEDICINE

Consensus Study Reports published by the National Academies of Sciences, Engineering, and Medicine document the evidence-based consensus on the study's statement of task by an authoring committee of experts. Reports typically include findings, conclusions, and recommendations based on information gathered by the committee and the committee's deliberations. Each report has been subjected to a rigorous and independent peer-review process and it represents the position of the National Academies on the statement of task.

Proceedings published by the National Academies of Sciences, Engineering, and Medicine chronicle the presentations and discussions at a workshop, symposium, or other event convened by the National Academies. The statements and opinions contained in proceedings are those of the participants and are not endorsed by other participants, the planning committee, or the National Academies.

For information about other products and activities of the National Academies, please visit www.nationalacademies.org/about/whatwedo.

PLANNING COMMITTEE ON ADVANCING GENE THERAPY FOR NERVOUS SYSTEM DISORDERS[1]

STORY LANDIS (*Co-Chair*), Director Emeritus, National Institute of Neurological Disorders and Stroke
LAMYA SHIHABUDDIN (*Co-Chair*), Sanofi
ZESHAN AHMED, Eli Lilly and Company
DAVID BREDT, Janssen Research & Development, LLC
DANIEL BURCH, PPD Biotech
JOSEPH BUXBAUM, Icahn School of Medicine at Mount Sinai
BEVERLY DAVIDSON, University of Pennsylvania Perelman School of Medicine
JOSHUA GORDON, National Institute of Mental Health
FRANCES JENSEN, University of Pennsylvania
JOHN KRYSTAL, Yale University
MARYANN REDFORD, National Eye Institute
TODD SHERER, The Michael J. Fox Foundation for Parkinson's Research
HAO WANG, Takeda Pharmaceuticals
CLINTON WRIGHT, National Institute of Neurological Disorders and Stroke

Health and Medicine Division Staff

CLARE STROUD, Director, Forum on Neuroscience and Nervous System Disorders
SHEENA M. POSEY NORRIS, Program Officer
PHOENIX WILSON, Senior Program Assistant
ANDREW M. POPE, Senior Director, Board on Health Sciences Policy

---

[1] The National Academies of Sciences, Engineering, and Medicine's planning committees are solely responsible for organizing the workshop, identifying topics, and choosing speakers. The responsibility for the published Proceedings of a Workshop rests with the workshop rapporteurs and the institution.

FORUM ON NEUROSCIENCE AND
NERVOUS SYSTEM DISORDERS[1]

---

[1] The National Academies of Sciences, Engineering, and Medicine's forums and roundtables do not issue, review, or approve individual documents. The responsibility for the published Proceedings of a Workshop rests with the workshop rapporteurs and the institution.

Reviewers

This Proceedings of a Workshop was reviewed in draft form by individuals chosen for their diverse perspectives and technical expertise. The purpose of this independent review is to provide candid and critical comments that will assist the National Academies of Sciences, Engineering, and Medicine in making each published proceedings as sound as possible and to ensure that it meets the institutional standards for quality, objectivity, evidence, and responsiveness to the charge. The review comments and draft manuscript remain confidential to protect the integrity of the process.

We thank the following individuals for their review of this proceedings:

JEAN BENNETT, University of Pennsylvania Perelman School of Medicine
VIVIANA GRADINARU, California Institute of Technology

Although the reviewers listed above provided many constructive comments and suggestions, they were not asked to endorse the content of the proceedings nor did they see the final draft before its release. The review of this proceedings was overseen by **ELI ADASHI,** Brown University. He was responsible for making certain that an independent examination of this proceedings was carried out in accordance with standards of the National Academies and that all review comments were carefully considered. Responsibility for the final content rests entirely with the rapporteurs and the National Academies.

Contents

1

Introduction and Overview[1]

Therapeutic development for brain disorders is entering its golden age, said Story Landis, co-chair of the Forum on Neuroscience and Nervous System Disorders of the National Academics of Sciences, Engineering, and Medicine. Among the most promising new therapeutic innovations are gene-targeted therapies.

After decades of scientific, clinical, and manufacturing advances, gene-targeted therapies have recently been approved for two rare monogenic neurological disorders: an inherited retinal disease caused by biallelic mutations in the *RPE65* gene (known clinically as some types of Leber congenital amaurosis or retinitis pigmentosa) and the progressive and often fatal neuromuscular disorder called spinal muscular atrophy. Gene-targeted therapies for many other neurological disorders are currently in development using several different technologies, said Lamya Shihabuddin, head of the genetic neurologic disease cluster in Sanofi's rare and neurologic diseases therapeutic area. These approaches include delivery of genes with viral or non-viral vectors, modulating or silencing gene expression with antisense oligonucleotides (ASOs), and other novel technologies on the horizon.

"The beautiful thing about gene therapy is that it makes everything, in theory, druggable," said Steven Hyman, director of the Stanley Center for

[1] The planning committee's role was limited to planning the workshop, and the Proceedings of a Workshop was prepared by the workshop rapporteurs as a factual summary of what occurred at the workshop. Statements, recommendations, and opinions expressed are those of individual presenters and participants; have not been endorsed or verified by the Health and Medicine Division of the National Academies of Sciences, Engineering, and Medicine; and should not be construed as reflecting any group consensus.

Psychiatric Research at the Broad Institute of the Massachusetts Institute of Technology and Harvard University. However, to move gene-targeted therapies from rare monogenic central nervous system (CNS) disorders to more common and complex diseases will require solving many technical challenges, said Shihabuddin. Among the challenges critical for success is robust and efficient delivery of gene-targeted therapies to specific regions of the brain and cell types. Other challenges she mentioned include working with regulators to move from first generation to second generation viral vectors that are safer and more potent, addressing issues of patient access and participation in clinical development, and sharing learnings and data from clinical studies. Addressing these challenges will require creativity and collaboration among academia, industry, research funders, regulators, and patients, said Shihabuddin.

Recognizing the need to bring this broad range of stakeholders together to address these issues, the Forum on Neuroscience and Nervous System Disorders convened a workshop titled Advancing Gene-Targeted Therapies for Central Nervous System Disorders in Washington, DC, on April 23 and 24, 2019.

WORKSHOP OBJECTIVES

The public workshop brought together experts and key stakeholders from academia, government, industry, philanthropic foundations, and disease/patient-focused nonprofit organizations to explore approaches for advancing the development of gene-targeted therapies for CNS disorders, and implications of developing these therapies. Participants explored lessons learned from both successful and unsuccessful clinical development programs; new knowledge about the genetic underpinnings of brain disorders; the current status and future potential of gene-targeted therapies for CNS disorders; challenges and potential solutions for translating preclinical findings to approved therapies; and patient and caregiver perspectives. They also discussed what will be needed to develop these therapies for common disorders such as Alzheimer's and Parkinson's diseases, as well as neuropsychiatric and neurodevelopmental disorders such as schizophrenia and autism. The workshop included approaches that target both DNA and RNA, as well as gene products using viral vectors, ASOs, and RNA interference. Box 1-1 presents the full Statement of Task and workshop objectives.

This field is evolving rapidly and the workshop could not cover all research and development under way in this domain, for example, preclinical and early clinical phase work targeting certain CNS disorders, such as forms of blindness other than that caused by biallelic *RPE65* mutations, Batten disease, and auditory disorders.

BOX 1-1
Statement of Task

An ad hoc committee will plan and conduct a 1.5-day public workshop that will bring together experts and key stakeholders from academia, government, industry, and nonprofit organizations to explore approaches for advancing the development of gene-targeted therapies for central nervous system (CNS) disorders, including approaches that target nucleic acids, such as adeno-associated viruses, antisense oligonucleotides, and RNA interference, as well as gene product-targeted therapies. Invited presentations and discussions will be designed to:

- Provide an overview of the current landscape of gene-targeted therapy approaches for CNS disorders.
- Discuss lessons learned from recent advances in gene therapy and antisense oligonucleotide development for retinal dystrophy and spinal muscular atrophy.
- Compare features of different gene-targeted therapy approaches in development for CNS disorders, and discuss how to match the approaches to specific diseases, addressing their respective administration, distribution, dose challenges, and potential long-term effects.
- Explore clinical development—including biomarker and clinical endpoint selection, trial design to demonstrate disease modification, and the regulatory path—for gene-targeted therapy approaches for rare genetic disorders that have more variable onset and progression.
- Discuss what it would take to move beyond rare genetic disorders to develop gene-targeted therapy approaches for common, heterogeneous disorders such as Alzheimer's and Parkinson's diseases.
- Explore opportunities for catalyzing development of gene-targeted therapy approaches for CNS disorders, including potential collaborative efforts among sectors and across disorders.

The planning committee will develop the agenda for the workshop, select and invite speakers and discussants, and moderate the discussions. A proceedings of the presentations and discussions at the workshop will be prepared by a designated rapporteur in accordance with institutional guidelines.

ORGANIZATION OF THE PROCEEDINGS

Chapter 2 describes the current landscape of and lessons learned from the development of gene-targeted therapies for CNS disorders, both approved therapies and those that have failed in clinical trials. Gene-targeted therapy approaches now in development and the challenges they face are explored in Chapter 3. Challenges related to the translation of gene-targeted therapy approaches from preclinical models to approved therapies are discussed in Chapter 4. Chapter 5 explores meaningful engagement of patients and families, as well as ethical issues related to the development and marketing of gene-targeted therapies, including issues related to data sharing and access. Advancing the development of gene-targeted therapies through further innovation and collaboration is discussed in Chapter 6.

2

Exploring the Current Landscape of Central Nervous System Gene-Targeted Therapies

Highlights

- The antisense oligonucleotide (ASO) medication nusinersen, which was the first Food and Drug Administration–approved drug to treat spinal muscular atrophy (SMA), demonstrates the potential of ASOs to treat genetically based central nervous system disorders (Bennett).
- In selecting an animal model for preclinical studies, it is critical that the model mimics the status of patients who will be enrolled in the study and that investigators understand the limitations of animal models (Kordower).
- The availability of naturally occurring large animal models of a genetic disease can expedite development of gene therapy by helping to define the dose range and magnitude and onset of treatment response, and to establish safety (Reape).
- Non-human primate models may help demonstrate that a treatment is capable of crossing the blood–brain barrier (Kaufmann).
- Natural history studies are critical to understand normal physiology and pathophysiology and to design efficient clinical programs (Bennett, Reape), but can be challenging to conduct in people with rare diseases (Kaufmann).
- In diseases with very severe effects such as SMA, treating patients as early as possible is important and may provide more robust effects (Bennett, Kaufmann).

- It is important to identify upfront what is a clinically meaningful change using both objective and subjective endpoints (Reape).
- When there is a risk involved in administering a therapy, it is important to define the trial population likely to benefit (Reape).
- It is important to engage and discuss with all experts—patients, families, patient advocacy groups, investigators, technical advisors, and regulators—and work with them throughout the development process starting in the early stages of development (Bennett, Reape).
- For gene therapies, durability of effect is crucial, so studies may need to be extended for several years (Reape).
- Most gene therapy trials have failed because of inadequate delivery of the gene to the appropriate target (Kordower).
- Many failed gene therapy trials are the result of investigators relying on animal models that do not accurately recapitulate the human disease, misinterpreting preclinical data, and lacking a clear understanding of the human disease and patient population (Kordower).

NOTE: These points were made by the individual speakers identified above; they are not intended to reflect a consensus among workshop participants.

Successful development of gene-targeted therapies for central nervous system (CNS) disorders over the past few years—particularly the approval of the antisense oligonucleotide (ASO) Spinraza® in 2016 for spinal muscular atrophy (SMA); Luxturna™ in 2017 for a rare form of inherited retinal dystrophy; and most recently in 2019, the gene replacement therapy Zolgensma® for the treatment of SMA[1]—were built on a long history of gene therapy products that were tested in clinical trials, but never made it to the clinic, said Lamya Shihabuddin. Lessons from both successful and unsuccessful trials are equally informative, said Shihabuddin.

APPROVED GENE-TARGETED THERAPIES FOR MONOGENIC CENTRAL NERVOUS SYSTEM DISORDERS

Single-gene or monogenic disorders, although each are relatively rare, offer perhaps the most straightforward approach for gene-targeted therapies. Indeed, said Biogen's Chris Henderson, the gene-targeted CNS therapies that have been successful so far have all targeted monogenic disorders in children.

---

[1] Zolgensma® was approved about 1 month after the workshop.

Starting with familial forms of disease makes sense because it allows investigators to work out how to design a modality to achieve the large effect sizes needed. The next step, he said, will be to find better targets for sporadic forms of disease and to move from treating childhood-onset to adult-onset disorders.

Nusinersen: An Antisense Oligonucleotide Treatment for Spinal Muscular Atrophy

In December 2016, the ASO medication nusinersen (Spinraza®) became the first Food and Drug Administration (FDA)-approved drug to treat SMA (Paton, 2017), a rare autosomal-recessive neuromuscular disorder and the leading genetic cause of infant mortality, caused by mutations or deletions in the survival motor neuron 1 (*SMN1*) gene, which encodes the SMN protein (Farrar and Kiernan, 2015). Nusinersen was approved by the European Medicines Agency (EMA) in June 2017.

C. Frank Bennett, senior vice president of research at Ionis Pharmaceuticals, used the approval of nusinersen as an example of the potential of ASOs to treat genetically based CNS disorders. Once synthetic ASOs bind to RNA, they can evoke different mechanisms to modulate its function, including degradation of the RNA, modulating splicing, or decreasing or increasing translation of a particular protein (see Figure 2-1). There are currently six approved antisense drugs on the market, said Bennett.

Mutation or deletion of *SMN1* causes a deficiency in production of the SMN protein, which results in motor neuron dysfunction. Late in human evolution, a duplication of *SMN1* resulted in a second gene called *SMN2*, which differs from *SMN1* by just 5 to 11 nucleotides, said Bennett. However, the *SMN2* gene has a change in one nucleotide within exon 7, which results in alternative splicing of the exon, with approximately 80 percent of transcripts skipping exon 7, which produces a truncated protein that is rapidly degraded. The remaining 20 percent of transcripts contain exon 7 and produce full-length, fully functional SMN protein.

SMA presents in a variable manner, said Bennett, ranging from type 1 infantile onset, which is associated with a very short life expectancy, to type 3 later onset, associated with a near-normal life expectancy. Disease severity correlates with the number of copies of the *SMN2* gene. Thus, most children with SMA type 1 have two copies of *SMN2*, begin to show symptoms before 6 months of age, and are never able to sit. Children with SMA type 2 usually have three copies of *SMN2*, begin to show symptoms after 6 months of age, are able to sit and stand but not walk, and have a shortened life expectancy. Children with SMA type 3 usually have three or four copies of *SMN2*, begin to show symptoms after 6 months of age, and have a near-normal life expectancy; although they may learn to walk, muscle weakness

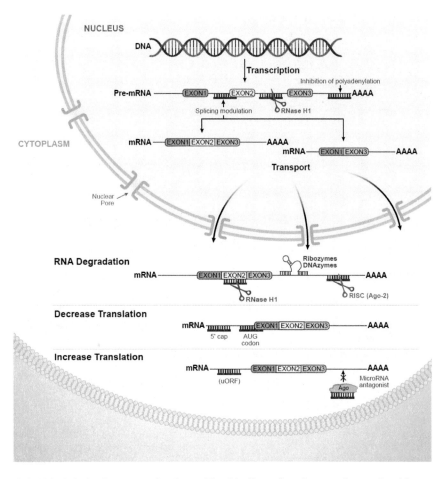

FIGURE 2-1 Antisense mechanisms. The binding of antisense oligonucleotides to the messenger RNA (mRNA) can result in degradation, decreased translation, or increased translation of the mRNA through different mechanisms.
SOURCE: Presented by C. Frank Bennett, April 23, 2019.

and skeletal deformities eventually lead to a non-ambulatory state for most of these children (Finkel et al., 2014; Rudnik-Schoneborn et al., 2009).

Nusinersen targets the *SMN2* pre-mRNA, binding to a sequence in the *SMN2* pre-mRNA, which modulates splicing and leads to production of full-length *SMN2* mRNA and *SMN2* protein (Hua et al., 2010). Preclinical studies established proof of mechanism and biology, determined the pharmacokinetic and pharmacodynamic relationship, optimized delivery methods, and demonstrated a lack of toxicity, said Bennett (Paton, 2017).

To design a clinical program, Bennett and colleagues (including partners at Biogen) relied on natural history studies published by the Pediatric Neuromuscular Clinical Research Network for SMA (Finkel et al., 2014; Kaufmann et al., 2012). These studies allowed them to demonstrate, for example, in an open-label Phase 2 study in infants with SMA type 1 that the survival benefit in patients treated with nusinersen differed markedly from the natural history of the disease and that benefits were greatest when infants were treated as early in the disease as possible, even before symptom onset (Finkel et al., 2016). Regulators were concerned, however, that these differences between study participants and natural history controls might reflect improved care of SMA patients or that healthier patients were being preselected for the study, he said. Thus, the sponsors designed a very large sham-controlled study. FDA acknowledges that an improvement in motor function scores instead of survival benefit might be acceptable, said Bennett. Fortunately, he said, the trial design included a prespecified interim analysis. This analysis showed that nusinersen improved both survival and motor function; these observations resulted in early termination of the trial (Finkel et al., 2017) and eventual approval by both FDA and EMA.

Voretigene Neparvovec: Gene Therapy for an Ultrarare Genetic Eye Disease

Kathleen Reape, chief medical officer at Spark Therapeutics, focused her presentation on clinical and regulatory challenges associated with the development of voretigene neparvovec (Luxturna®), a gene therapy product approved by FDA in 2017 and EMA in 2018 for the treatment of an ultrarare inherited retinal disease caused by biallelic mutations in the *RPE65* gene. *RPE65* encodes an enzyme necessary for production of a vitamin A derivative in photoreceptors (Bennett et al., 2012). The absence of a functional enzyme leads to the buildup of toxic precursors, the death of photoreceptors, and progressive loss of vision. Voretigene supplies a copy of the gene encoding the enzyme and restores the visual cycle, said Reape.

One of the early decisions the developers made was to base the indication on a molecular diagnosis rather than clinical symptoms, because even though the hallmark feature of the disorder is nyctalopia, or night blindness, only individuals specifically with biallelic *RPE65* mutations will benefit from the therapy, said Reape. Requiring a molecular diagnosis led to certain hurdles in terms of participant recruitment and enrollment for clinical trials given the limited availability of genotyping. This continues to be a challenge for the commercial product, she said.

Development of voretigene benefited from the availability of a naturally occurring large animal model of the condition—the Briard dog—and extensive preclinical work by Jean Bennett and colleagues at the University of Pennsylvania (Bennett et al., 2012; Bennicelli et al., 2008). The dogs enabled definition of the dose range for the first clinical trial and provided insight into the expected magnitude and onset of the treatment response, said Reape. Other challenges to overcome in the development of voretigene included balancing the potential benefit of the treatment with the risk of surgical delivery via subretinal injection in children, the selection of primary and secondary endpoints, and the choice of a control group.

Individuals with biallelic *RPE65* mutations progressively lose the ability to detect light, resulting in impaired navigation and other vision-dependent activities (Chung et al., 2018). Because existing functional vision tests were found to inadequately capture the effect of illumination on speed and accuracy of navigation, investigators developed and validated a novel endpoint—the multiluminance mobility test (MLMT)—which tests functional vision and incorporates components of visual field, visual acuity, and light sensitivity, said Reape (Chung et al., 2018). The MLMT tests the performance of participants navigating a course with obstacles and arrows to follow at seven different light levels with a minimum number of errors in a prespecified amount of time. The primary endpoint was the mean change in lowest passing light level. Reape said the investigators created 12 different standardized courses that were presented in a randomized fashion to minimize learning effects. They used an independent reading center with two masked adjudicators using a detailed grading protocol with clearly defined parameters for what constituted errors, passes, and fails. Secondary endpoints included full-field light sensitivity threshold testing, monocular MLMT performance, and visual acuity, as well as exploratory endpoints assessing visual fields, she said, adding that participants or parents also completed a visual function questionnaire to assess activities of daily living relevant to vision loss (Russell et al., 2017a). Reape noted the importance of including both subjective and objective endpoints for these types of studies to ensure that any change measured is clinically meaningful.

Choosing a control group for this trial was complicated, said Reape. Often for ultrarare diseases, natural history data can be used; however, such data did not exist for this condition. Using the contralateral eye was also considered, but raised concerns that in developing children, leaving one eye untreated could cause other problems or that the rate of degeneration may not be symmetrical in the two eyes, leading to incorrect conclusions. In addition, in the real-world setting, each eye would be dosed separately within a relatively short period of time. Reape said the final decision was to use a two-to-one randomization, have the untreated control group observed for 1 year, and then offer control subjects the opportunity to cross over and receive this treatment. Because the trial included young children, the company rejected the idea of using a sham surgical procedure; thus, the trial was an open-label (unmasked) study. Results from the original untreated control group after crossing over and receiving treatment confirmed that the magnitude and onset of the treatment effect was similar among participants (see Figure 2-2).

In these trials of rare conditions that enroll such small numbers of participants, capturing a meaningful incidence of adverse events is difficult, said Reape. She also noted that the labeling reflects the difficulty of separating out adverse events caused by the product versus the administration procedure, vitrectomy, and subretinal injection, adding that when there is a risk associated with the administration procedure, it is especially important to identify the population that is likely to benefit.

AVXS-101: Clinical Phase Gene Replacement Therapy for SMA

Another gene-targeted treatment for SMA was described by Petra Kaufmann, vice president, research and development translational medicine at AveXis.[2] AVXS-101 (Zolgensma®) is a gene replacement therapy product designed to treat the root cause of SMA by targeting the mutation in *SMN1*, said Kaufmann. AVXS-101 delivers the gene via a vector constructed from the adeno-associated virus 9 (AAV9), which is able to cross the blood–brain barrier and reach motor neurons in the spinal cord. Inside the AAV9 capsid shell, a double-stranded piece of DNA has been created from the relevant parts of the transgene controlled by a promoter that enables sustained production of the missing *SMN1* protein and flanked by inverted terminal repeats, which accelerate transcription of the transgene and production of a full-length functioning protein (Powell et al., 2015) (see Figure 2-3).

Kaufmann cited preclinical studies in a mouse model of SMN that showed a dose-dependent increase in survival when treated with an AAV9-SMN construct (Foust et al., 2010), and another study in newborn-to-3-year-old cynomolgus macaques demonstrating that AAV9 injected into the cerebrospinal fluid crosses the blood–brain barrier and delivers its transgene to motor neurons, resulting in restricted expression of the gene in the central nervous system (Bevan et al., 2011). Another study in a pig model of SMA showed that presymptomatic treatment with AAV9-SMN prevented the development of SMA symptoms (Duque et al., 2015).

These preclinical studies led to a Phase 1 clinical trial in 15 infants with SMA1, with 3 patients receiving a low dose and 12 receiving the intended higher dose (Mendell et al., 2017). The primary outcome was safety; a secondary efficacy outcome was survival free of permanent ventilation by Bilevel Positive Airway Pressure for more than 16 hours per day, and an exploratory outcome was a decline on the Children's Hospital of Philadelphia Infant Test for Neuromuscular Disorders motor function scale (Finkel et al., 2014).

---

[2] This therapy was approved by FDA in May 2019, approximately 1 month after the workshop.

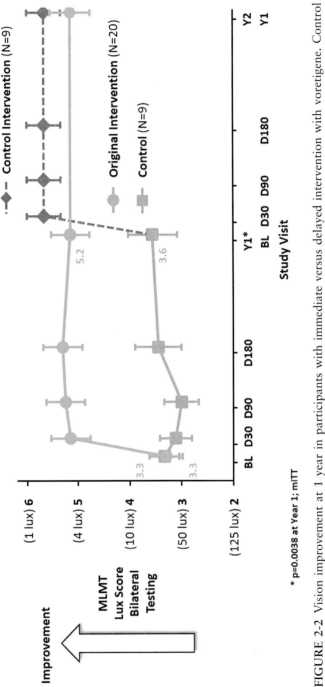

FIGURE 2-2 Vision improvement at 1 year in participants with immediate versus delayed intervention with voretigene. Control participants who began receiving voretigene at the end of the 1-year study period quickly achieved the same level of vision improvement as measured by the multiluminance mobility test (MLMT) as those in the intervention group who received voretigene at the beginning of the trial.

SOURCES: Presented by Kathleen Reape, April 23, 2019; Russell et al., 2017a,b.

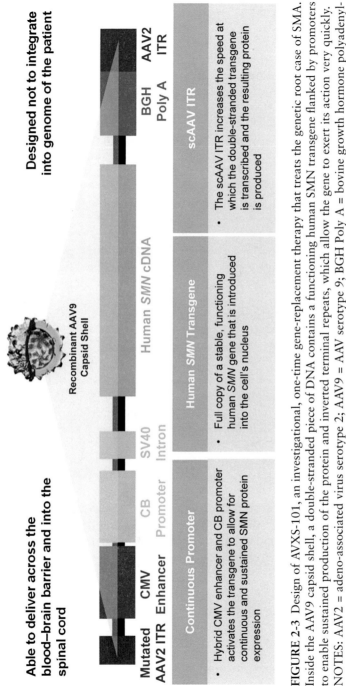

FIGURE 2-3 Design of AVXS-101, an investigational, one-time gene-replacement therapy that treats the genetic root case of SMA. Inside the AAV9 capsid shell, a double-stranded piece of DNA contains a functioning human SMN transgene flanked by promoters to enable sustained production of the protein and inverted terminal repeats, which allow the gene to exert its action very quickly.
NOTES: AAV2 = adeno-associated virus serotype 2; AAV9 = AAV serotype 9; BGH Poly A = bovine growth hormone polyadenylation; CB = chicken β-actin; cDNA = complementary DNA; CMV = cytomegalovirus; ITR = inverted terminal repeat; scAAV = self-complementary AAV; SMA = spinal muscular atrophy; SMN = survival motor neuron; SV = simian virus.
SOURCE: Presented by Petra Kaufmann, April 23, 2019.

Natural history data were used as a control. Kaufmann noted the difficulty of conducting natural history studies in patients with rare and serious diseases such as SMA. "It's a real gift of altruism on the part of families to participate over often more than a year in a study when there is no treatment," she said. She credited not only the families, but also the SMA Foundation for funding the Pediatric Neuromuscular Clinical Research Network study, and the National Institute of Neurological Disorders and Stroke for funding the National Network for Excellence in Neuroscience Clinical Trials SMA Infant Biomarker Study, which enrolled and for 24 months followed 26 infants with genetically confirmed SMA and 27 age, sex, and birthweight-matched healthy infants. Among the SMA cohort, 12 died and 2 received invasive ventilatory support (Kolb et al., 2017).

Kaufmann briefly described the large effect size observed in the Phase 1 study: 11 of the 12 patients who got the proposed dose could sit briefly, and some even walked. At the long-term follow-up, they had not lost milestones, and some had even gained. The demonstrated safety as well as transformative improvements on efficacy endpoints led to a multicenter Phase 3 trial. Kaufmann said that interim data from this Phase 3 study demonstrated improved survival and motor function improvement. On May 24, 2019, FDA approved Zolgensma® as the first gene therapy to treat children younger than age 2 with SMA (FDA, 2019).

Kaufmann noted that the clinical studies also showed that younger patients, some of them presymptomatic, did better than older patients. Even those less than 6 weeks old with two or three copies of the mutated *SMN2* gene, that is, those predicted to have a severe form of SMA, did well, suggesting that the greatest benefit is in patients treated early. The lesson learned from this observation, she said, is the importance of early diagnosis so that patients can be treated as early as possible.

One patient in the Phase 3 study made good progress in terms of motor function but, sadly, died from SMA. Kaufmann described how the parents provided an altruistic gift by consenting to an autopsy, which provided a unique opportunity to investigate biodistribution of the vector. This case study showed that, similar to what has been seen in animal studies, the vector was broadly distributed in all tissues evaluated, including all regions of the spinal cord. SMN expression was also demonstrated in motor neurons of this patient, she said.

UNSUCCESSFUL GENE THERAPY TRIALS: LESSONS LEARNED

In efforts to identify an effective treatment for Parkinson's disease (PD), Jeffrey Kordower, the Alla V. and Solomon Jesmer Professor of Aging and Neurological Sciences at the Rush University Medical Center, has conducted several gene therapy and cell replacement trials, all of which have failed.

Although disappointing, Kordower said these trials have also provided valuable lessons relevant to ongoing and future gene-targeting trials.

In the late 1990s, Kordower and colleagues used intracerebroventricular injections of glial-derived neurotrophic factor (GDNF) to treat a man with PD (Kordower et al., 1999). The treatment not only failed to improve the man's parkinsonian symptoms, but also was associated with substantial side effects. Kordower said the trial was not supported by preclinical data and never should have been performed. Poor distribution of GDNF in the brain indicated that a better delivery method was needed. Indeed, Kordower said that most gene therapy trials fail because of delivery problems.

Next, they tested a gene therapy approach using GDNF delivered by a lentiviral vector to monkeys that had been given injections of 1-methyl-4-phenyl-1,2,3,6-tetrahydropyridine, a neurotoxin that induces degeneration of nigrostriatal neurons and motor deficits similar to those seen in patients with PD (Kordower et al., 2000). While these animals improved far more than control animals, and a subsequent Phase 1 human trial showed adequate safety and tolerability, a Phase 2 trial failed. Kordower said the reason is that progression of PD results from a combination of brain pathologies (Buchman et al., 2019). Reversing nigrostriatal dysfunction alone is not sufficient, he said.

A subsequent trial of a different neurotrophic factor called neurturin also failed, said Kordower. Inadequate delivery of the agent to the brain again was the culprit, although this time the reason was that in order to avoid a long surgical procedure, the investigators injected too low of a dose of the protein to the brain. There was also another problem. As shown originally by Patrick Aebischer, Christophe Lo Bianco, and colleagues in 2004, GDNF has no beneficial effect in a synucleinopathy model of PD (Lo Bianco et al., 2004), said Kordower. He and his colleagues showed in a recent autopsy study that even patients with prodromal PD have nerve fibers filled with α-synuclein (Chu et al., 2018). There was no way this approach was going to work, said Kordower.

Kordower said the failures of GDNF trials illustrate the multiple points where development of gene-targeted therapies can go wrong. First, he cautioned that preclinical data can be misleading. Because animals do not develop PD in nature, the models used in preclinical studies may not accurately reflect the disease process in humans. Preclinical studies, he said, should be designed not to be successful, but to inform clinical trials so that those trials will be successful. He argued that many failed clinical trials are the result of translational scientists moving forward without a clear understanding of the human disease or the patient population they are trying to treat. Finally, he stressed the importance of interpreting data with rigor and honesty. Adhering to these guidelines will save time and money while not compromising the safety of trial participants, he said.

3

Gene-Targeted Therapy Approaches for Central Nervous System Disorders: Opportunities and Challenges

Highlights

- Gene-targeted therapies include those that target RNA or DNA and either a gene itself or a modulator of that gene (Davidson).
- The safety of chronic expression versus redosing or regulated expression is an important consideration when targeting RNA (Davidson).
- When targeting DNA, the delivery modality should match the biodistribution goal of the therapy (Davidson).
- Challenges to the development of gene-targeted therapies for central nervous system (CNS) disorders include whether the gene should be delivered to the brain itself or peripherally, blood–brain barrier penetration, and the potential to elicit an immune response (Crystal, DeVos).
- More work and better models are needed to determine whether immunosuppression is necessary, when to immunosuppress, and with what drugs (Crystal).
- Oligonucleotide therapeutics, including antisense oligonucleo-tides and small interfering RNAs, can be designed to enhance pharmacokinetic properties, potency, duration of effect, and stability (Khvorova).
- Adeno-associated virus is the most widely used viral vector for gene therapy, but is limited by its capsid capacity and pre-existing antibodies (Samulski).

- Although gene-targeted therapies for CNS disorders have focused mostly on monogenic disorders, there has been progress in developing them for common, complex polygenic disorders as well (Abeliovich).
- For loss-of-function disorders, cross-correction may sometimes provide sufficient gene expression even if transduction efficiency is low (Abeliovich, Davidson).
- CRISPR/Cas gene editing approaches are being developed to treat gain-of-function disorders such as Huntington's disease (Davidson).

NOTE: These points were made by the individual speakers identified above; they are not intended to reflect a consensus among workshop participants.

Central nervous system (CNS) therapies historically have been restricted to small molecules because large molecules do not get into the brain very well, said David Bredt, global head of neuroscience discovery at Johnson & Johnson Pharmaceutical Group. The field has tried to develop monoclonal antibodies for neurological diseases, but thus far has been unsuccessful, he said. Gene therapy offers an alternate way of selecting CNS targets, but as noted by Jeffrey Kordower in Chapter 2, delivery of gene-targeted therapies to their targets has proved challenging. New technologies that incorporate novel capsid proteins and/or carefully selected promoters are in development to ensure that therapies are expressed in the cells of interest in the CNS, said Bredt.

When choosing the appropriate modality, several issues need to be considered, said Beverly Davidson, director of the Raymond G. Perlman Center for Cellular and Molecular Therapeutics at the Children's Hospital of Philadelphia and professor of pathology and laboratory medicine at the Perelman School of Medicine, University of Pennsylvania. Whether targeting RNA or DNA, the delivery approach must be chosen with safety in mind, said Davidson. For example, the safety of chronic expression versus redosing or regulated expression is an important consideration when targeting RNA. When targeting DNA and RNA, the delivery modality should match the biodistribution goal of the therapy, or redosing may need to be considered. Whether targeting the genome or RNA with sustained delivery, Davidson noted the importance of considering immune responses. Genome editing raises additional safety considerations, including consideration of what happens at the editing site.

For gene addition approaches, Davidson noted the importance of fitting the genetics to the therapy being developed, that is, determining whether the optimal target is the gene itself or a modifier of the gene. Other considerations include the region or cell type to be targeted, and for loss-of-function disorders, whether cross-correction—the ability of non-transduced cells to take up genetically modified gene products through receptor binding—can be exploited. She added that the tolerability of gene products also needs to be addressed, with expression fine-tuned if a gene product is not well tolerated.

DELIVERY OF GENE-TARGETED THERAPIES TO THE CENTRAL NERVOUS SYSTEM

Sarah DeVos, project leader at Denali Therapeutics, described three different modalities for delivery of gene-targeting therapeutics to the CNS:

- Naked gene therapy, where the genetic material is delivered without a viral capsid to modulate where the gene is expressed.
- Peripheral adeno-associated virus (AAV) gene therapy, in which the vector delivers its cargo to a peripheral organ such as the liver, where the gene is expressed and protein generated and could be secreted.
- Central AAV gene therapy, where the vector delivers the gene via direct injection into the brain or intravenously if the vector is capable of crossing the blood–brain barrier.

Blood–brain barrier penetration is a hurdle for both naked gene therapy and peripheral approaches, said DeVos. However, she has shown that both the naked gene therapy approach with antisense oligonucleotides and the central approach with AAV have potential for repressing the expression of the microtubule-associated protein tau gene, more commonly referred to simply as tau, one of the two hallmark pathogenic proteins in Alzheimer's disease and several other forms of dementia known as tauopathies.

Gene-targeted therapies and immunotherapies also have the potential to elicit an immune response from the person being treated, which can reduce the efficacy of a treatment, particularly if redosing is needed. Ronald Crystal, professor and chair of the department of genetic medicine at the Weill Medical College of Cornell University, said more work and better models are needed to determine whether immunosuppression is necessary, when to immunosuppress, and with what drugs.

ASO Therapies

DeVos demonstrated in mouse models expressing mutant human tau that repressing tau expression with antisense oligonucleotides (ASOs) reversed tau pathology (DeVos et al., 2017). One advantage of this ASO approach, she said, is that because it is not permanent, its safety can be assessed even if the full biological function of a protein is not fully understood.

Anastasia Khvorova, professor in the RNA Therapeutics Institute at the University of Massachusetts Medical School, said that for oligonucleotide therapeutics, safe delivery to the CNS can also be achieved by defining the chemical and structural architecture of the oligonucleotide to have the desired pharmacokinetic properties, that is, absorption, distribution, metabolism, and excretion. Once this structural backbone has been defined, the oligonucleotide can be easily reprogrammed with different sequences to silence genes on demand.

This design approach has been used to generate three types of oligonucleotide therapeutics that are currently in clinical development, said Khvorova (Khvorova and Watts, 2017) (see Figure 3-1). The simplest type, called steric-blocking oligonucleotides, simply bind to mRNA to block translation or alter slicing. Spinraza®, the only approved oligonucleotide therapy in the CNS, is an example of a steric-blocking antisense product. The second class of antisense compounds described by Khvorova require interaction with the enzyme ribonuclease H to cleave the targeted RNA and downregulate gene activity. RNA interference (RNAi), the most complex type of oligonucleotide therapeutic, interacts with other cellular proteins to form the RNA-induced silencing complex and silence gene expression.[1] Over the past two decades, Khvorova said the chemistry has evolved substantially to enhance the pharmacokinetic and pharmacodynamic properties of small interfering RNAs (siRNAs), increase their potency and duration of effect, and chemically stabilize the oligonucleotides without interfering with their protein machinery interactions.

In August 2018, patisiran became the first RNAi-based therapeutic to receive Food and Drug Administration (FDA) approval.[2] Although the drug treats a peripheral rather than CNS disease (polyneuropathy), Akshay Vaishnaw, president of research and development at Alnylam Pharmaceuticals, Inc., used it as a case study to exemplify what has been learned about RNAi in the clinic. The lessons learned from the development of patisiran can be applied to the development of RNAi for CNS diseases, he said. The Phase 3 studies of patisiran showed first that RNAi can be used to suppress a target for long periods of time, and that this translates into neurological benefit in patients, said Vaishnaw. The drug not only halted progres-

---

[1] For an overview of RNA interference (RNAi), see https://www.umassmed.edu/rti/biology/how-rnai-works (accessed August 9, 2019).

[2] FDA News Release, August 10, 2018: FDA approves first-of-its-kind targeted RNA-based therapy to treat a rare disease. See https://www.fda.gov/news-events/press-announcements/fda-approves-first-its-kind-targeted-rna-based-therapy-treat-rare-disease (accessed June 6, 2019).

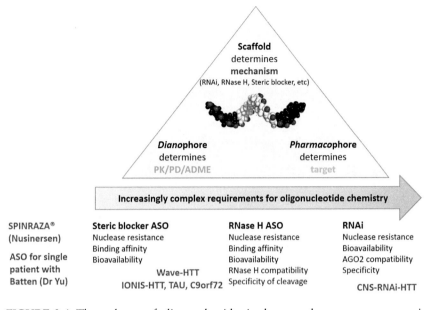

FIGURE 3-1 Three classes of oligonucleotides in the central nervous system: anti-sense oligonucleotides (ASOs) can modulate RNA expression through one of three different mechanisms determined by the chemical structure and composition of the scaffold.

NOTES: ADME = absorption, distribution, metabolism, and excretion; ASO = anti-sense oligonucleotide; PD = pharmacodynamics; PK = pharmacokinetics; RNAi = ribonucleic acid interference; RNase H = ribonuclease H.

SOURCE: Presented by Anastasia Khvorova, April 23, 2019.

sion of disease, but was also associated with improvement in a composite neuropathy score that assesses symptoms across several sensory and motor domains. He noted that the drug was also well tolerated with an acceptable safety profile.

Because oligonucleotides do not cross the blood–brain barrier in healthy adults, they need to be delivered directly to the cerebral spinal fluid either by intrathecal or intracerebroventricular (ICV) injection or by implantation of an Ommaya reservoir, said Khvorova. Her lab has developed RNAi oligo-nucleotides that get robustly distributed throughout the brain after a single ICV injection. In a Huntington's disease (HD) mouse model, ICV injection of a siRNA directed against the mutant huntingtin gene (*HTT*) demon-strated significant protein silencing for up to 6 months, said Khvorova. Yet, while silencing huntingtin protein expression in a mouse model is exciting, the human brain is much larger and more diverse. Because of this, her lab has been working with two larger animal models: sheep and non-human primates. In both models, they have shown that a single ICV injection of siRNA results in widespread delivery throughout the cortex and distribution to deep brain structures. Most importantly, a single ICV injection of siRNA efficiently silenced huntingtin protein expression in the cortex and deep brain structures of non-human primates, said Khvorova.

Vaishnaw and colleagues are developing another approach, which they call a conjugate-based approach, to target siRNAs to the CNS. To target the liver in the development of patisiran, they used N-acetylgalactosamine as the ligand, conjugated to an siRNA that targets mutant forms of the transthyretin gene (Adams et al., 2018). For delivery to the CNS, they have identified other novel ligands conjugated to siRNA targeting *SOD1* (superoxide dismutase 1, a gene implicated in familial amyotrophic lateral sclerosis) or β-catenin (used as a control). In rat models, they demonstrated dose-dependent protracted and reversible silencing of these genes following a single or multiple dose delivered intrathecally, said Vaishnaw. He added that while siRNAs are known to be cleared rapidly from the CNS, the conjugated siRNAs have far superior uptake by neuronal tissues relative to unconjugated siRNAs or to ASOs. They have also tested this approach in non-human primates with similar results, including uptake in all key cell types of the CNS (neurons, microglia, and astrocytes).

Viral Delivery of Gene Therapy

Two FDA-approved gene therapy products, Luxturna and Zolgensma, use a viral vector—AAV—to deliver therapeutic genes to their targets, and while many other viruses have been used for gene therapy applications, AAV remains the most widely used (Lundstrom, 2018). The first approval of an AAV gene therapy product—Glybera—in 2012 opened the floodgates of funding for development of gene therapies and has enabled the field to flourish, said Robert Kotin, scientific founder of Generation Bio and adjunct professor at the University of Massachusetts Medical School. Currently several different serotypes of AAV are being used as vectors in gene therapy clinical trials, said Kotin. All are derived from non-pathogenic dependoparvoviruses, which have proven to be safe and effective in numerous clinical trials. They vary in terms of tissue specificity, transduction efficiency, and antigenicity (Rayaprolu et al., 2013).

According to R. Jude Samulski, co-founder of the AAV gene therapy company AskBio and former director of the University of North Carolina Gene Therapy Center, AAV gene therapies are defined by four characteristics: (1) the capsid, which determines what cells to target; (2) the transgene, which can be altered and optimized for better translation; (3) the promoter, which regulates gene transcription; and (4) the mode of production. Petra Kaufmann added that what goes into the engineering and design of viral vectors is largely empirical. It requires finding a promoter that provides a certain tropism and the appropriate level of expression, she said.

Challenges associated with AAV therapeutics include the limited capsid capacity and preexisting and cross-reacting neutralizing antibodies, which limit dosing to a single administration, said Samulski. Switching the *formulation* of a therapy by switching serotypes or genetically modifying the capsid may provide superior vectors. For example, using directed evolution, which is discussed further in Chapter 6, vectors have been developed that selectively cross the seizure-compromised blood–brain barrier and transduce cells in the CNS (Gray et al., 2010). This approach could be used to deliver gene therapy for seizure disorders, said Samulski.

In their efforts to develop therapies that would repress production of tau, DeVos and colleagues are developing a longer lasting central gene therapy approach by packaging into an AAV capsid a zinc finger protein fused to a transcription factor that recognizes and represses tau. She said they hope to couple this with an AAV variant called AAV-PHP.B. PHP.B is a capsid protein that more efficiently transduces neurons after intravenous injection in rodents (Challis et al., 2019; Deverman et al., 2016). Recent developments on engineered capsids are described in Chapter 6.

To determine the biodistribution of an AAV vector in vivo, Crystal and colleagues have developed a non-invasive technique by covalently labeling the AAV capsid with a positron emitter that can be detected using positron emission tomography. In non-human primates, they have shown that intravenously administered vectors home primarily to the liver, but also to the bone marrow. Even following direct injection into the brain, some of the vectors travel to the bone marrow and liver, said Crystal. In animals that were hyperimmunized (to mimic a person with preexisting immunity), they showed that when the vector was readministered several months later, nearly all of the vector homed to the spleen. This kind of information could be important clinically because it can help assess whether immunosuppression should be used before, during, or after administration of gene therapy, said Crystal.

IDENTIFYING THERAPEUTIC TARGETS

Gene-targeted therapies for CNS disorders discussed thus far have focused primarily on monogenic disorders; however, there has also been progress in developing gene-targeted approaches for more common complex polygenic disorders such as Parkinson's disease (PD). Dopaminergic therapies currently available for PD address motor symptoms of disease, but do not impact disease progression, said Asa Abeliovich, founder and chief executive officer of Prevail Therapeutics. However, PD is not just a motor disease. Non-motor symptoms, which often become dominant and lead to the most serious morbidity, are not the result of dopaminergic neuron loss in the mid-brain, said Abeliovich. To have meaningful disease modification requires thinking about PD as a brain-wide disease, he said.

For more than 100 years it has been known that intracellular protein inclusions called Lewy bodies are the main pathological finding in PD, which suggested that lysosome dysfunction may be a core mechanism underlying the disease, said Abeliovich. Genetic studies since then have identified many PD-associated genes that play a direct role in lysosome function and trafficking, he said (Abeliovich and Gitler, 2016). One of these is the glucocerebrosidase gene, *GBA1*. *GBA1* mutations cause the lysosomal storage disorder Gaucher disease and are the most common genetic risk factors for PD (Sidransky et al., 2009), affecting all aspects of PD including severity and age of presentation, progression, and risk of progression to dementia, said Abeliovich. For example, mutations in *GBA1* increase the likelihood that a patient will progress to cognitive dysfunction and dementia. He added that there is a range of severity associated with the more than 300 known *GBA* mutations and a gene dosage effect such that homozygotes have more aggressive cognitive decline than heterozygotes (Liu et al., 2016a). Even mutations in just one copy of *GBA1* are associated with an increased risk of PD, said Abeliovich.

Several different gene therapy approaches have been developed for Gaucher disease, said Abeliovich. A lentiviral vector used to transduce hematopoietic stem cells with the GBA gene was shown to prevent Gaucher disease progression in mouse models (Dahl et al., 2015). Abeliovich said that while this vector is not delivered efficiently to the brain, the study showed that through cross-correction, transduction of only about 10 percent of the cells drove sufficient GBA expression to correct symptoms. AAV vectors delivering *GBA1* to the CNS have also been shown to lower α-synuclein levels in synuclein transgenic mice (Sardi et al., 2013), and intravenous injection of AAV-PHP.B-GBA1 prevented formation of α-synuclein inclusions in PD mouse models (Morabito et al., 2017).

Davidson noted that the capacity for cross-correction is not universal. When designing gene therapies intended to take advantage of cross-correction, one must first determine whether the gene products are well secreted and well tolerated. Beautiful cross-correction has been achieved for several different lysosomal storage diseases, she said, but some gene products need to be reengineered for better secretion. If the gene products are well secreted, they may have deleterious effects. For example, in the Davidson laboratory, an attempt in mouse models to advance gene therapy for progranulin deficiency by cross-correction with AAV9 showed that expressing progranulin elicited massive T cell infiltration and disappearance of the hippocampus (Amado et al., 2019). This raises the question of whether overexpressing other proteins in other diseases could have untoward effects and whether this problem could be dealt with by turning protein expression off or expressing the protein in a pulsatile manner, said Davidson. For secreted proteins, these questions need to be answered in a stepwise fashion, she said.

Most of the therapies discussed this far are intended to treat loss-of-function disorders. For gain-of-function disorders, other challenges must be considered, said Davidson. She focused her comments on microsatellite expansion disorders in which short sequences of nucleotides are repeated up to 1,000 times in coding or non-coding regions of the genome (Gao and Richter, 2017). More than 40 disorders are caused by microsatellite expansions, including HD, spinocerebellar ataxia, Fragile X disease, and many others, said Davidson.

Targeting the DNA in these disorders by editing out the toxic gain-of-function gene presumably could represent a one-and-done approach. She and her colleagues are developing CRISPR/Cas[3] gene editing approaches to treat HD. To develop this approach, they needed to consider how, where, and when to intervene and what part of the gene to target. Given that HD progresses over 15 to 20 years with massive degeneration of the basal ganglia and cortical structures, Davidson and colleagues concluded that the treatment should be initiated very early in the disease course, while there were still cells left to treat. Selecting which part of the gene to target was informed by earlier research by Gillian Bates and colleagues, who showed that the toxic form of the *HTT* protein results from aberrant splicing of exon 1 in mutant *HTT* (Sathasivam et al., 2013). More recently, Laura Ranum and colleagues showed that repeat expansions can be translated in both the sense and antisense directions, and that the resulting proteins (called repeat-associated non-ATG, or RAN proteins) are very toxic (Banez-Coronel et al., 2015). These findings suggested to Davidson that the entire length of the mutant expanded allele should be deleted.

An investigator in her laboratory, Alex Monteys, answered the question of how to intervene, said Davidson. He devised a CRISPR strategy that took advantage of single nucleotide polymorphisms linked to the mutant allele, but not present on the normal allele so that he could selectively edit out only the *HTT* gene that contained the mutation, leaving the non-mutated *HTT* gene intact to carry out its normal functions (Monteys et al., 2017). This enabled him to dramatically reduce the levels of mutant *HTT* mRNA and protein levels in injected areas of the brain in HD mouse

---

[3] Clustered Regularly Interspaced Short Palindromic Repeats (CRISPR) and CRISPR-associated (Cas) genes provide an efficient, accurate, rapid, and inexpensive method for genome editing. To learn more about CRISPR-Cas, see https://www.broadinstitute.org/files/news/pdfs/PIIS0092867415017055.pdf (accessed June 3, 2019).

models. Davidson's lab has also demonstrated the ability to silence the locus using a novel approach called CRISPR interference.

To advance these approaches, Davidson said more efficient methods are needed to improve delivery of the therapies to larger brains (e.g., with lipid nanoparticles) or alternatively, to improve the safety of virally delivered editing machinery.

4

Translating Gene-Targeted Therapies from Bench to Bedside

Highlights

- The availability of large animal models has enabled the successful development of gene-targeted therapies for several diseases, including Duchenne muscular dystrophy (Samulski).
- Non-human primate models may be predictive of safety and efficacy in humans (Bennett).
- Innovations in clinical trial design, such as leveraging historical control data and adapting a trial based on interim data, may enable more efficient trials needing fewer participants (Panzara).
- Natural history studies and patient registries are critical enablers of clinical trial recruitment for life-threatening and rare diseases (Panzara, Sampaio, Vaishnaw).
- Balancing risks and benefits will differ depending on disease-specific factors, such as whether a condition is aggressive or slowly progressive (Kaufmann, Kordower, Reape).
- Regulatory agencies have established expedited development programs that can be applied to gene-targeted therapies for serious and rare conditions (Kjeken, Marks).
- Drug development for complex polygenic disorders is especially challenging and requires different regulatory pathways, including those designed to evaluate combination therapies (Marks, Sampaio).

- Large effect sizes for gene therapy may mitigate the challenges of identifying clinically meaningful and measurable outcomes when trials are small, the clinical readout is long, or there are no reasonably similar surrogates (Sampaio).
- Regulatory pathways are needed to enable bridging studies from first to second generation viral vectors and from one disorder to another (Samulski, Vaishnaw).
- Vector production for non-clinical and clinical studies is difficult and expensive and thus requires collaborative efforts from academic, industry, and regulatory scientists (Kotin, Marks).

NOTE: These points were made by the individual speakers identified above; they are not intended to reflect a consensus among workshop participants.

In his opening remarks for the session on translation, moderator Daniel Burch, global medical officer at PPD Biotech, echoed earlier remarks about the excitement and fast-moving nature of the gene-targeted therapy field, and characterized working in this area during the past few years as "drinking from a fire hose."

R. Jude Samulski showed videos of two boys with Duchenne muscular dystrophy (DMD) who participated in clinical trials of a gene therapy treatment. DMD is a rare, fatal, X-linked genetic disorder caused by mutations in the dystrophin gene that prevent production of dystrophin, a protein essential for normal muscle function. Samulski said that within months of receiving the gene therapy by IV infusion, the boys progressed from not being able to climb steps to playing Little League baseball. The videos he showed illustrate what can happen when a technology developed in the laboratory is successfully translated to humans and what some of the challenges are. For example, asked Beverly Davidson, what happens when new vectors are developed that appear to be 10 times more efficient than the old vectors? Should trials of the old vectors be discontinued and replaced by trials of the new vectors, or can they be phased in gradually? What kind of bridging studies will be required to ensure safety?

ENABLING TRANSLATION WITH PRECLINICAL MODELS

Chapter 3 described Akshay Vaishnaw's early work to develop conjugated small interfering RNAs as a therapeutic modality for central nervous system (CNS) disorders. To optimize the pharmacology of the compounds in development, he and his colleagues have initiated studies to understand the correct dose and frequency in animal models, with a goal of achieving therapeutic levels with dosing every 6 months or annually. Other ongoing Investigational New Drug (IND)-enabling studies are exploring the distribution of the conjugates and gene knockdown in particular cell types as well as identifying novel ligands that exert knockdown only in specific cell types within the CNS. While cell models can be useful translational tools, animal models are especially important for CNS disorders, said Anastasia Khvorova. Particularly for psychiatric and neurodegenerative disorders, most cell models are non-predictive because they do not adequately model the complex infrastructure and environment in which cells function in the brain, she said.

In contrast with many other disease areas, a major translational bottleneck for psychiatric disorders is the limited availability of appropriate predictive models for both efficacy and toxicity, said Steven Hyman. Indeed, the successful gene-targeting approaches described in Chapter 2 were enabled in part by the availability of large animal models, both naturally occurring (inherited retinal disease) and genetically engineered (spinal muscular atrophy, or SMA) models. Samulski described how the golden retriever muscular dystrophy model—a model derived from dogs identified in the early 1980s with spontaneous dystrophinopathies and an X-linked pattern of inheritance (Kornegay, 2017)—was used to test an adeno-associated virus (AAV)-mediated gene therapy approach to a deficiency in dystrophin protein. For example, he showed photographs of one of these dogs who, after receiving a sufficient dose of the vector, lived a normal dog's life and actually had increased muscle mass. More importantly, said Samulski, the dog displayed a good safety profile. Frank Bennett noted that in developing gene-targeted therapies for SMA, non-human primates were used only to study biodistribution and safety because humans are the only species to have the alternate *SMN2* gene. Large animal models also allow preclinical studies to represent the effects of aging on uptake and distribution of vectors or antisense oligonucleotides, noted Lamya Shihabuddin.

While primate models may be most predictive because they are evolutionarily closer to humans, Jeffrey Kordower noted that the immune response of primates or their response to immunosuppressive drugs is highly variable. In addition, he said, little is known about the receptors for AAV vectors in different species.

CLINICAL TRIAL DESIGN CHALLENGES
FOR GENE-TARGETED THERAPIES

In designing clinical trials, sponsors must make decisions regarding inclusion and exclusion criteria, endpoints, controls, and balancing risks and benefits. Bennett added that sponsors must also consider the natural progression of the disease, the patient population available for a clinical trial, and the anticipated effect size of the drug. Kathleen Reape agreed, noting that the trial design will differ for a fatal debilitating condition compared to a slowly progressive disease. Chris Henderson added that one treatment may not be fully efficacious for all patients.

Michael Panzara, chief medical officer at Wave Life Sciences, Ltd., described the clinical program for survodirsen, a potential treatment for boys with DMD. Survodirsen is designed to restore functional dystrophin through the method of exon skipping, which enables production of a shorter but functional protein (Kole and Krieg, 2015). Based on a favorable safety and tolerability profile established in a recently completed Phase 1 single ascending dose study enrolling 40 boys, a Phase 2/3 study is now being planned, he said. In addition, boys who completed the Phase 1 study are eligible for an open-label extension study at a dose expected to lead to exon skipping, said Panzara. Data from this study are expected later in 2019, including assessment of dystrophin expression in muscle biopsy, and are intended to comprise an important component of the company's submission for accelerated approval, he said.

Running in parallel, the Phase 2/3 study called DYSTANCES 51, set to begin in July 2019, was selected by the Food and Drug Administration (FDA) for its Complex Innovative Trials Designs pilot program,[1] an initiative under the 21st Century Cures Act, said Panzara. Among the innovative trial design features planned for DYSTANCES 51 is the leveraging of historical control data to help augment the placebo arm. This approach is intended to reduce the number of participants required to deliver conclusive efficacy results, minimize the number of participants in the placebo treatment arm, and accelerate the study program, he said. A second key innovation is the use of Bayesian repeated measure modeling to adapt the trial based on interim dystrophin analyses, said Panzara. Simultaneously, they will develop a Bayesian disease progression model, which will incorporate historical control data and interim biopsy data to predict the probability of success and potentially to adjust enrollment in an ongoing fashion to improve the efficiency of the trial.

Panzara noted that the historical control data are being contributed by several companies that have conducted DMD clinical trials. The Critical Path Institute will assist in this process as a neutral convener, housing the datasets for those who would prefer that the data sit with a third party. The modeling work and placebo data collected in this trial will be shared with the field to leverage learnings and propel the field forward. Panzara

---

[1] For more information about FDA's Complex Innovative Trial Designs Pilot Program, go to https://www.fda.gov/drugs/development-resources/complex-innovative-trial-designs-pilot-program (accessed June 7, 2019).

added that he hoped this would serve as a model for future rare disease clinical trials.

The innovations in clinical trial design described by Panzara address the significant recruitment and retention challenges sponsors face when conducting clinical trials for life-threatening disease. These challenges are exacerbated for rare diseases, where access to patient populations is critical but may be limited, said Vaishnaw. Natural history studies may provide access to potential trial participants, and patient registries have been developed in several disease areas to improve the efficiency of recruitment. For example, in the Huntington's disease (HD) space, the CHDI Foundation developed a platform called ENROLL-HD,[2] which has been running for more than 6 years and has 20,000 participants, said Cristina Sampaio, chief medical officer at the CHDI Foundation and professor of clinical pharmacology at the University of Lisbon. Registries have helped fuel translation in other disease areas as well. Vaishnaw said that in DMD, the size of the population has allowed several registries to prosper, collect meaningful data, and provide an important resource for academia and industry. For micro-orphan diseases, however, he said that competing registries in both academia and industry can be a significant impediment to the drug development process.

The selection of clinically meaningful endpoints will differ depending on the condition and the population affected, said Reape. For example, in establishing what constituted a clinically meaningful change in the novel endpoint developed for the voretigene studies (discussed in Chapter 2), the investigators had to consider the real-world meaningfulness of restoring vision in children compared with adults who have been blind since birth, she said. Vaishnaw added that appropriate endpoints and biomarkers are particularly difficult to identify for rare diseases for which natural history studies are so difficult.

Balancing risks and benefits and establishing minimal effect sizes will also differ depending on other disease-specific factors, such as whether a condition is fatal and debilitating or slowly progressive, said Reape. Kordower agreed, noting that it may be appropriate to accept smaller benefits in certain subpopulations in which the disease is especially aggressive. In early-stage trials when there is a lot of uncertainty, risks are higher so the potential benefit to trial participants should also be high, said Petra Kaufmann. Kordower added that safety and tolerability studies are typically underpowered to answer efficacy questions and cautioned sponsors not to try to assess efficacy from a safety and tolerability study. However, Henderson suggested that efficacy data from a safety and tolerability study, if appropriately interpreted, can speed up the progress of a trial.

---

[2] For more information about ENROLL-HD, go to https://www.enroll-hd.org (accessed June 17, 2019).

Reape noted that the *RPE65* gene therapy trials included detailed responder analyses to try to determine if characteristics such as age influenced response. There were two participants who showed no change in performance (improvement or decline) on the multiluminance mobility test, she said, but they were unable to identify any single underlying characteristic that both had in common. However, they learned from the natural history study that age is a very loose indicator of retinal degeneration, with a high degree of individual variation, as would be expected with a progressive disease. Because the treatment requires the presence of viable retinal cells, surrogate markers such as retinal thickness and visual field were used to assess retinal viability, although she noted that those tests do not directly assess retinal function.

REGULATORY PATHWAYS

Gene therapies fall into the regulatory category of advanced therapy medicinal products, which also includes cell therapies and xenotransplantation, said Peter Marks, director of the Center for Biologics Evaluation and Research (CBER) at FDA. He added that gene therapies for serious conditions are eligible for several of FDA's expedited development programs, including Fast Track, Priority Review, Accelerated Approval, Breakthrough Therapy, and Regenerative Medicine Advanced Therapy (RMAT). RMAT became law as part of the 21st Century Cures Act at the end of 2016 to expedite gene and cell therapies, tissue engineering products, and certain combination approaches, he said. To get this designation, the product must address a serious or life-threatening disease or condition and there must be preliminary evidence of its potential to address an unmet medical need. RMAT-designated products may also be eligible for priority review and accelerated approval, Marks noted. In the past 2-plus years, Marks said 33 products—mostly cellular or cell-based gene therapy products—have been granted this designation.

To help advance the development of gene and cell therapies, Marks said FDA has also issued several guidance documents, taken steps to reduce the administrative burden of regulatory approval, established several clinical development and manufacturing initiatives, and helped develop standards. He also mentioned the INitial Targeted Engagement for Regulatory Advice on CBER producTs (INTERACT) program,[3] which enables sponsors to meet with FDA for a non-binding, relatively informal pre-IND meeting to discuss preclinical, manufacturing, and clinical issues related to therapies in early stages of development.

---

[3] For more information about the INTERACT program, see https://www.fda.gov/vaccines-blood-biologics/industry-biologics/interact-meetings-initial-targeted-engagement-regulatory-advice-cber-products (accessed June 8, 2019).

The European Medicines Agency (EMA), though organized quite differently from FDA, functions in a similar manner, according to Rune Kjeken, scientific director for advanced therapies at the Norwegian Medicine Agency and a member of EMA's Committee for Advanced Therapy and the Scientific Advice Working Party. Structured as a network of regulatory agencies from the 28 European Union member states plus Iceland and Norway, the work of EMA is conducted by scientific committees and working parties, said Kjeken.

Like FDA, EMA is responsible for assessment and decision making at all steps of the regulatory pathway, including final marketing approval, said Kjeken. Also like FDA, EMA writes guidelines, including disease-specific and modality-specific (e.g., gene therapy) guidelines. EMA also has a program similar to INTERACT, which is called the Innovation Task Force.[4] Approval of clinical trials, however, remains with the competent authorities of individual nations, he said.

EMA also has an early access mechanism called PRIME (PRIority MEdicines), similar to what FDA calls "breakthrough designation," to foster development of medicines with high public health potential, said Kjeken. Since December 2018, he said, about 50 products have been accepted into the PRIME program, about 20 of which are gene therapy products.

Kjeken said EMA has a procedure for parallel scientific advice with FDA. It also works in parallel with health technology assessment bodies to ensure that consideration is given to the potential value of a new drug and how it will perform in the real world. Kjeken predicted this will become increasingly important in coming years as the more drugs developed for rare diseases exert an ever-greater impact on overall health care costs.

Matching Modalities and Regulatory Pathways to Specific Disorders

Regulators evaluate gene-targeted therapies differently from more traditional pharmacological therapies for several reasons, including the invasiveness of the interventions, the durability of effect, and issues related to placebo controls and participant recruitment, according to Sampaio. For the treatment of CNS disorders, the invasiveness of gene therapy approaches is somewhat more acceptable than for systemic disorders, she said, because of the 20-year history of using deep brain stimulation as a treatment approach for Parkinson's disease (PD); however, intravenous delivery would represent a major step forward over intrathecal administration.

For complex polygenic disorders where the pathophysiology of the disease is not fully understood, drug development is even more challeng-

---

[4] For more information about EMA's Innovation Task Force, see https://www.ema.europa.eu/en/documents/leaflet/innovation-task-force_en.pdf (accessed June 8, 2019).

ing, said Marks. Sampaio agreed, adding that while combination therapy is widely believed to be necessary to treat neurodegenerative diseases, regulators have been reluctant to embrace these approaches. Nonetheless, she said, there is a combination gene therapy product called ProSavin that is currently being tested in clinical trials for the treatment of PD (Palfi et al., 2018). Using a lentiviral vector, ProSavin delivers genes for three enzymes involved in the biosynthesis of dopamine.

Clinical trials for gene-targeted therapies are often constrained by the small number of potential participants, even in non-rare diseases, because not everyone will be a candidate for gene therapy, particularly if there is invasive administration, said Sampaio. Small numbers of participants and the severity of the condition being treated may also lead sponsors to propose alternatives to placebo-controlled trials. However, Sampaio argued that while placebo controls in very small trials may not produce the statistical power to demonstrate efficacy, they can nevertheless ensure blinding. This is important to avoid safety misreporting and to facilitate a balanced interpretation of biomarkers, keeping in mind that even biochemical markers can change with placebo. The need for using a sham intervention as a placebo may also add logistical constraints, she said.

Identifying appropriate and clinically relevant outcomes may also be challenging, particularly if the clinical readout is long or there are no reasonably like surrogates, said Sampaio. She argued, however, that the potential for very large effect sizes from gene therapy—even possible cures—may mitigate some of these problems, particularly those that result from the necessity of conducting trials with small numbers of participants. Although the potential of having a durable effect increases the appeal of gene therapy, it can be difficult to prove, she said.

Transitioning from First to Second Generation Vectors

In January 2019, a statement from Peter Marks and Scott Gottlieb, then FDA Commissioner, predicted that by 2020, FDA would be receiving more than 200 IND applications per year and that by 2025, they would be approving 10 to 20 cell and gene therapy products per year.[5] Samulski expressed concern that with this "tsunami of therapeutics" coming forward at a time when the technology is in the midst of a shift from first to second generation technologies, drug developers might be unwilling or

---

[5] Statement from FDA Commissioner Scott Gottlieb, M.D., and Peter Marks, M.D., Ph.D., director of the Center for Biologics Evaluation and Research on new policies to advance development of safe and effective gene therapies. See https://www.fda.gov/news-events/press-announcements/statement-fda-commissioner-scott-gottlieb-md-and-peter-marks-md-phd-director-center-biologics (accessed June 5, 2019).

unable to take advantage of superior vectors because only the inferior first generation vectors have been fully evaluated, endorsed, or approved by regulators. He suggested that developers and regulators will need to work together to craft strategies for bridging studies that will enable an efficient shift from one *formulation* to another even as that change in *formulation* may affect the specificity of targeting, the immune response to the capsid, payload size, transduction efficiency, and need for repeat dosing. Vaishnaw added that regulatory pathways are also needed that would enable quick bridging studies from one disorder to another, given that the platforms for developing therapies hold much in common even when designed for different conditions.

MANUFACTURING CAPACITY

The best vectors in the world are useless if they cannot be manufactured in sufficient quantities, said Robert Kotin. Thus, a major challenge for gene therapy drug development is chemistry, manufacturing, and control, he said, noting that vector production for both non-clinical and clinical vectors is difficult and expensive. Moreover, while relatively small doses are needed for subretinal injections to treat ocular indications, other CNS gene therapies may require much larger doses depending on the delivery method and indication. For example, systemic dosing for the treatment of diseases such as DMD require relatively large doses, said Kotin.

Over the past two decades, methods of producing AAV vectors have evolved to enable large-scale production of vectors at good manufacturing practice (GMP) facilities, said Kotin. Collaboration between academic researchers and industry has been critical to this evolution, he said. For example, a partnership between the University of Massachusetts Medical School (UMMS) and industry partners brought together the expertise of virologists and vectorologists at UMMS with the industry's engineering expertise to generate the large quantities of good laboratory practice vectors needed to support large-animal, dose-escalation studies. These processes may then be transferred to a GMP facility for large-scale manufacturing.

Developing and delivering gene therapies to the many patients with rare diseases will only be possible if manufacturing costs can be driven down to a sustainable level for common diseases with a big market potential, added Marks. Thus, he said, FDA's efforts to streamline manufacturing are especially important. A commonality among all advanced therapy medicinal products is that product quality, safety, and efficacy are inextricably linked, he said. Thus, he noted that for these products a controlled manufacturing process and an understanding of critical quality attributes is essential. Manufacturing AAV vector products, for example, requires dealing with multiple manufacturing challenges, including empty capsids, purification, and contaminating nucleic acids, he said, adding that only a few companies have mastered this process to date. He suggested that the translation of scientific advances made in academic laboratories to commercially manufactured products that help patients could be advanced by developing a set of non-proprietary AAV vectors and a "cookbook" of how to engineer vectors that could transfer easily into proprietary systems.

5

Meaningful Engagement of
Patients and Families

Highlights

- Zeal and enthusiasm for gene therapy can lead investigators to overlook warning signals observed in preclinical and clinical studies, and to therapeutic misconception among trial participants (Bennett, Kaufmann, Sampaio, Tabor).
- Meaningful engagement of patients and families has been embraced by funders and advocacy organizations as essential to the successful and ethical development of innovative treatments, including gene-targeted therapies (Coetzee, Landis, Sampaio, Tabor).
- Understanding patients' and caregivers' values and attitudes about benefits, risks, and side effects can help providers and investigators communicate more effectively with patients about treatment decisions (Tabor).
- Many patients are willing to share their data in order to advance science; they also want more information about risks, and they want access to their data (Tabor).
- Neutral parties such as the Critical Path Institute can provide the infrastructure for data sharing that protects the interests of patients and investigators (Panzara).
- With many new gene-targeted therapies on the horizon and their high costs threatening to overwhelm the health care sys-

tem, analyzing cost effectiveness and developing innovative pricing approaches have become essential (Tabor).

NOTE: These points were made by the individual speakers identified above; they are not intended to reflect a consensus among workshop participants.

Zeal and enthusiasm underlie some of the ethical dilemmas raised by gene therapy, according to Holly Tabor, associate professor of medicine at the Stanford University School of Medicine and associate director for clinical ethics and education at the Stanford Center for Biomedical Ethics. She cited the case of 18-year-old Jesse Gelsinger, who died in 1999 from a severe immune reaction to the gene therapy treatment he received as part of a Phase 1 clinical trial for the metabolic disorder ornithine transcarbomylase deficiency (Sibbald, 2001). Tabor quoted Robert Steinbrook, M.D., who wrote,

> In their zeal to help patients with a life-threatening disease, leading researchers at one of the premier academic medical centers in the United States lost their focus. They overlooked warning signals suggesting that the experimental intervention was not safe, with tragic, fatal consequences. (Steinbrook, 2008, p. 117)

The case provides lessons that resonate with other emerging and innovative treatments, said Tabor. These lessons relate to inclusion criteria, recruitment, therapeutic misconception, informed consent, transparency, conflict of interest, and institutional oversight, she said. The Gelsinger case also highlighted the need to strengthen and improve regulatory structures, maximize safety, and consider carefully who should be in a Phase 1 trial; create systems that prevent conflicts of interest; and increase transparency around all stages of clinical trials, said Tabor. She suggested that these challenges can be addressed by conducting empirical analysis of informed consent procedures for gene therapy trials, interviewing participants and researchers about their views on some of these ethical issues, and developing and testing shareable tools to mitigate therapeutic misconception and optimism.

Cristina Sampaio agreed that participants' expectations resulting from therapeutic misconception need to be carefully managed. Therapeutic misconception can be defined as existing

> when individuals do not understand that the defining purpose of clinical research is to produce generalizable knowledge, regardless of whether the

[participants] enrolled in the trial may potentially benefit from the intervention under study or from other aspects of the clinical trial. (Henderson et al., 2007, p. 1736)

As treatments become more complex and invasive and as more hype is generated for a treatment, participants and families may convince themselves that a cure is possible only if they do everything possible, including disrupting their lives, to gain access to a trial. She noted that strategies have been identified that can reduce therapeutic misconception (Christopher et al., 2017).

One way to avoid therapeutic misconception, said Petra Kaufmann, is to communicate transparently with patients and patient groups. Frank Bennett echoed her comment, adding that it is important for parents to recognize that this is a team effort in which their participation is essential. His team has found that when parents are more proactive in caring for their children and dealing with the complications of spinal muscular atrophy (SMA), the children actually do better.

FACILITATING PATIENT AND FAMILY ENGAGEMENT

Meaningful engagement and shared governance with patients and families is important, said Tabor, and requires more than including them on advisory boards. Rather, it requires learning about their lived experiences with their conditions without assuming they all have the same perspective and attitudes. Timothy Coetzee, chief advocacy, services, and research officer at the National Multiple Sclerosis Society, agreed, noting that patient perspectives and attitudes are evolving with regard to participation in placebo-controlled trials, sharing data with others and gaining access to their own data, and switching treatments. Patients are moving from passive to fully activated, he said, and dealing with the consequences of that activation requires moving from a recruitment mindset to an engagement mindset.

Sampaio said that in the United Kingdom, sponsors are required to submit their clinical trial protocols to a formal committee populated only by patients with different types of diseases in order to get approval. The committee comments on the protocol and may recommend changes. She added that a voluntary international committee called the HD Coalition for Patient Engagement (HD-COPE) is also available to review and make recommendations regarding Huntington's disease (HD) protocols and research plans.[1]

---

[1] For more information about HD-COPE, see https://ehma.org/2018/05/14/multi-act-kicks-off-today-bringing-research-closer-patients-society (accessed June 10, 2019).

Coetzee noted that the European Union has funded the MULTI-ACT project[2]—with leadership provided by the Italian Multiple Sclerosis Society—with a broad spectrum of partners to advance the science of patient input and foster engagement of all stakeholders in the development of new tools to assess, from multiple perspectives, the value and impact of research and innovation on people with brain diseases. He observed that MULTI-ACT has developed a particularly useful construct for patient engagement involving four domains: inform, involve, consult, and co-design. While the end goal is to develop safe and effective treatments, Coetzee said it is also important to ensure affordable access, which will require embracing all stakeholders and not simply leaving decision making to policy makers.

Tabor said the Patient-Centered Outcomes Research Institute is another model of how funding agencies have tried to mandate and facilitate patient engagement. The old models of patient engagement through patient and advocacy groups have strengths to build on, she said, but new approaches such as those that incorporate social media are also needed. Jill Morris, a program director at the National Institute of Neurological Disorders and Stroke (NINDS), added that the National Center for Advancing Translational Sciences requires data coordinating centers in the Rare Diseases Clinical Research Network to have an engagement and dissemination core to promote better engagement of industry and advocacy groups.

Characterizing and understanding patients' and caregivers' values around treatment decisions can help providers communicate more effectively about benefits, risks, side effects, and eligibility criteria for a trial, according to Tabor. She recommended that clinicians engage patients in explicit discussions about their awareness, knowledge, and potential misinformation about the natural history of the disease as well as their values and goals. For example, when she and her colleagues interviewed adults and parents of children with SMA about pursuing treatment with nusinersen, they found that patients and parents were trading off values and priorities when they assessed risks and benefits (Pacione et al., 2019). While one parent believed the potential benefits were insufficient to balance against the predicted continual decline in quality of life, an adult with SMA believed the drug would help her maintain a certain level of independence despite the barriers and challenges she faced. One mother believed the repeated intrathecal injections and a life focused around hospitals would conflict with their family's goal to help their child to not feel disabled.

Patient inclusion is important at all levels, not just for clinical trials and treatment decisions, said Story Landis. She recalled that when NINDS

---

[2] For more information about MULTI-ACT, see https://ehma.org/2018/05/14/multi-act-kicks-off-today-bringing-research-closer-patients-society (accessed June 10, 2019).

was planning programs for Parkinson's disease that required better metrics and initiatives, patients and families were more satisfied with the initiatives and efforts once they were brought into the discussions. Registries and natural history studies can promote engagement as well as enable clinical trials, added Daniel Burch. However, maintaining registries so they remain relevant for clinical trials can be challenging, said Sampaio, because diseases progress as participants age. For ENROLL-HD, mentioned in Chapter 4, a complex mathematical model has been created to guide future enrollment in the registry so that in 5 years, they will continue to have trial-ready participants, she said. The problem of multiple competing registries, which Akshay Vaishnaw mentioned in Chapter 4, also exists for non-rare diseases. Coetzee said there are 20 multiple sclerosis registries with some 60,000 participants, all started by various investigators. Although federating the data might be possible, the value of doing so is unclear because it would probably cost tens of millions of dollars, he said.

Patients' Views on Data and Information Sharing

Data sharing is an additional challenge and one in which registry and clinical trial participants want to play a more active role, said Tabor. Although many patients are willing to share data in order to advance science, they want complete information about risks and to be informed about their individual results when the trial ends, rather than having to wait until the Food and Drug Administration (FDA) has approved a treatment, she said. She added that trial participants should be more engaged in decisions companies make about sharing placebo and non-placebo arm data with the field, which may require building new strategies for getting informed consent. Michael Panzara mentioned that neutral parties such as the Critical Path Institute can provide the infrastructure for data sharing in a manner that protects the interests of companies and academic researchers as well as the confidentiality of patients.

Patients and parents are increasingly getting their information through social media rather than from their physicians, said Tabor. Trial participants who post online about the process of getting injections and other aspects of a trial have in some cases unblinded themselves, she said. Tabor and colleagues found that patients and families found this information to be more reliable, useful, and up to date than the information obtained from other sources. From these social media groups, they also obtained useful information about insurance coverage, social support, reducing social isolation, obtaining medical equipment, and other important issues, she said.

Tabor suggested that new frameworks are needed to identify and address ethical challenges associated with gene-targeted therapies, rather than addressing ethical issues on a case-by-case basis. Lessons from systems set up in California for governance of stem cell research could provide a model pathway, she said. These lessons include making room for laypeople in governance structures, promoting transparency, minimizing secrecy, creating opportunities for learning and innovation, and building alliances and collaboration among stakeholders, said Tabor (Mintrom and Bollard, 2009).

ACCESS, COST, AND EQUITY

The high costs of gene-targeted therapies pose additional ethical challenges related to access and allocation of scarce resources, said Tabor, noting that many of these challenges are neither new nor unique to gene-targeted therapies. Indeed, she said, in the early 1960s, perhaps the first-ever bioethics committee was established at a Seattle hospital to help determine who would get the very limited slots for dialysis (Jonsen, 2007). The high cost of admission to intensive care units has also been investigated for many years, said Tabor, yet there are few processes for deciding where, when, and how patients should be admitted. She suggested that if all or even a few of the gene therapies currently in the pipeline are approved, issues of costs and access will become even more critical.

The approvals of Glybera, Spinraza, and Zolgensma illustrate many of these challenges, said Tabor. In 2012, after a very long development and approval process, Glybera was approved in Europe as a treatment for lipoprotein lipase deficiency with a requirement for post-marketing surveillance. At a cost of about $1 million per patient, 60 people were dosed in European trials, but only 1 patient paid for the treatment. The drug was withdrawn in the United States and not pursued in Europe, said Tabor. Spinraza was approved by FDA in 2016 at an estimated cost of $750,000 for the first year and $350,000 annually for the rest of the patient's life. Tabor said that insurance coverage has been variable, and although Biogen offers financial assistance for Spinraza, there are many reports in the media of patients having difficulty with access. Zolgensma is predicted to cost more than $2 million, but will only require one treatment. All three of these drugs treat rare diseases, which somewhat mitigates the impact of the high costs at least at a societal level, but gene-targeted therapies are on the near-term horizon for many more common diseases such as hemophilia, sickle cell anemia, and macular degeneration, said Tabor. If 20 to 25 new gene therapies are approved each year over the next few years, as Peter Marks and others anticipate, the costs could overwhelm the health care system. Moreover, said Tabor, the costs related to gene-targeted therapies are occurring in a landscape of societal concerns about increased overall costs of drugs and medical care.

An independent, nonprofit research institution, the Institute for Clinical and Economic Research (ICER),[3] produces reports analyzing the effectiveness and value of drugs and other medical services and shares their findings with the public, payers, and industry in an attempt to stimulate informed public discourse on the topic, said Tabor. She noted, however, that ICER has been criticized by patient groups and others because they are partially funded by industry and for how they assess cost effectiveness. These groups claim that payers use ICER's findings to deny patients access to drugs, said Tabor.

Referring to a recent article about value-based pricing for emerging gene therapies (Garrison et al., 2019), Tabor suggested that there are elements of value that are not well assessed for rare, debilitating, or life-threatening diseases. These elements include the severity of the disease, equity, and the value of hope. While ICER and other groups typically assess value based on cost per quality-adjusted life-year (QALY), survey research suggests that people view QALY gains differently for different subpopulations, said Tabor. For example, people generally give priority to subpopulations with poor baseline health, including those at the end of life, she said. In response to public criticism, ICER issued a statement in December 2018 saying they would no longer depend solely on QALYs, but would also include a measure called "equal value of life years gained" (evLYG), which incorporates incremental gains in length of life regardless of changes in quality of life. Thus, a treatment that adds 1 year of life for the most severely affected patients would receive the same evLYG as one that adds 1 year of life for healthier people.

ICER also published an evidence report on the effectiveness and value of Spinraza and Zolgensma for the treatment of SMA (ICER, 2019). According to Tabor, ICER concluded that while both treatments improve the lives of patients and families, the cost of Spinraza far exceeds the threshold that would make it cost effective. They called for Novartis/AveXis to set a lower launch price for Zolgensma than the hypothetical $4–$5 million price that had initially been floated.

Several innovative approaches to pricing for these very expensive therapies have been proposed, said Tabor (Kaltenboeck and Bach, 2018). Value-based pricing, for example, sets the price based on the magnitude of benefit. Another approach treats the price like a mortgage, where the insurer agrees to pay the cost over time. Yet another requires the manufacturer to refund the cost of the treatment when an agreed-on outcome is not met. Tabor said that while these approaches may not have the kinds of effects needed, they demonstrate that efforts are being made to address the difficult issue

---

[3] For more information about the Institute for Clinical and Economic Review, go to https://icer-review.org (accessed June 14, 2019).

of pricing. However, her research suggests that more attention also needs to be paid to the impact of costs on the person who is experiencing the condition. Access and equity are key, she said. She asserted that scientists, policy makers, and clinicians have a moral and ethical responsibility to make sure that gene therapy and other innovative approaches are not only available to the very wealthy or highly insured. Patient and stakeholder engagement will be key to ensuring that issues of equity are considered, she said.

6

Future Directions in the Development of Gene-Targeted Therapies

Highlights

- Non-viral gene transfer using closed-end linear duplex molecules offer the potential to transduce cells without triggering an immune response, but brain disorders would require direct injection into the central nervous system (Kotin).
- Small molecules that modulate splicing have shown promise in correcting the mutations that cause spinal muscular atrophy, Huntington's disease, and familial dysautonomia (Bhattacharyya).
- Nanocapsules composed of biodegradable polymers and containing the ribonucleoproteins needed for CRISPR/Cas9 genome editing can be targeted to specific cells to achieve rapid editing with low off-target effects (Gong).
- Directed evolution techniques applied to the development of adeno-associated virus (AAV) vectors have resulted in vectors that cross the blood–brain barrier in rodents (Gradinaru).
- Intracellular antibodies (intrabodies) delivered with an AAV vector have prevented aggregation and promoted clearance of α-synuclein in rat models (Kordower).
- To tackle challenges in delivering gene-targeted therapies to specific targets, the expertise of synthetic biologists, systems biologists, computational biologists, and scientists with expertise in computational fluid dynamics will be needed (Gradinaru, Suh).

- Cross-disciplinary collaborations are needed to translate novel technologies from rodents to non-human primates (Gradinaru).
- Developing gene therapy applications for common neuro-psychiatric and neurodevelopmental disorders is particularly challenging because they are highly polygenic (Hyman).
- Highly penetrant genes associated with neurodevelopmental disorders may represent targets for gene therapy (Buxbaum).
- The non-coding portion of the genome may be as targetable as the genes that encode proteins (Davidson, Hyman, Khvorova).
- Pre-competitive partnerships among companies and academic researchers could expedite development of gene-targeting therapies and extend the scope of these therapies to more diseases (Crystal, Henderson, Kaufmann, Koroshetz).

NOTE: These points were made by the individual speakers identified above; they are not intended to reflect a consensus among workshop participants.

Although most of the successful and unsuccessful studies discussed at this workshop focused on monogenic diseases, Chris Henderson suggested that going forward, it will be important to use learnings from these familial forms to find targets for treating sporadic and non-monogenic disorders. To achieve this goal while also advancing gene-targeted therapies for monogenic disorders will require technological innovation as well as attention to the safety of new approaches and a clearer understanding of which approaches are appropriate for specific diseases and targets, said Lamya Shihabuddin. Frances Jensen, professor and chair of neurology at the Perelman School of Medicine, University of Pennsylvania, added that it will also be important to consider how to coordinate implementing new discoveries in the clinic. The cancer field has been facing this challenge for decades, she said, as one new modality eclipses another. While trying to do what is best for patients by offering them the most advanced therapies, clinicians have at the same time had to consider the fact that there may be something even better in the pipeline, she said.

NEW TECHNOLOGIES ON THE HORIZON

As described in Chapter 3, viral vectors currently dominate the pipeline of gene-targeted therapies. Yet, Robert Kotin said that even as there are continuing efforts to find new and better vectors, other technologies are also advancing rapidly.

Non-Viral Methods

Kotin described a novel approach to gene transfer that delivers only the DNA of interest (the gene), flanked by inverted terminal repeats from the adeno-associated virus (AAV), that forms closed-end, linear duplex molecules (CELiD). Compared to bacterial plasmids, which have also been used for non-viral gene transfer, CELiD DNA has no prokaryotic modifications that might trigger an innate immune response and no endotoxins, said Kotin. He and his colleagues have produced close-ended DNA (ceDNA) constructs with the gene for green fluorescent protein or nuclear-localized β-galactosidase, and showed that following transfer by hemodynamic injection into the tail vein of mice, gene expression was constant over 7 days (Li et al., 2013). Adding a liver-specific promoter to the construct resulted in fairly constant gene expression in liver tissue over 10 weeks and essentially no change in CELiD copy number, said Kotin. More recently, investigators have demonstrated efficient transduction in the central nervous system (CNS) using ceDNA constructs delivered directly to rat brain using convection-enhanced delivery. One advantage of the ceDNA approach is that the vectors are produced using a good manufacturing practice-compatible process, said Kotin. However, optimizing the chemistry for specific tissue targeting remains a challenge in developing ceDNA methodologies, and it will not be possible to target the CNS with systemic delivery, he said.

Small Molecules to Modulate Splicing

Small molecules that modify post-transcriptional processing of RNA represent yet another novel therapeutic approach for genetic disorders, according to Anuradha Bhattacharyya of PTC Therapeutics, which has developed a platform to discover and develop small molecule splicing modifiers that are orally available and have broad tissue distribution. They are currently applying this technology to the development of treatments for spinal muscular atrophy (SMA), familial dysautonomia (FD), and Huntington's disease (HD), said Bhattacharyya.

The SMA therapeutic in development targets endogenous *SMN2* with a small molecule splicing modifier that promotes the inclusion of exon 7, said Bhattacharyya. Two other strategies are also being pursued, she said. Each of these approaches provides many potential druggable targets, said Bhattacharyya. One approach corrects splicing mutations in pre-mRNA; this strategy is being used to enable inclusion of an exon that is usually skipped in the disease setting of FD. The other approach being pursued as a treatment for HD activates a pseudo-exon in the huntingtin gene pre-mRNA, which creates a premature stop codon, resulting in degradation of the mRNA and protein. In HD mouse models, Bhattacharyya said they have demonstrated a dose-dependent decrease in huntingtin protein across all relevant brain areas following oral delivery of the compound.

Nanoplatforms for Brain-Targeted Genome Editing

CRISPR/Cas9 genome editing, mentioned in Chapter 3, is a powerful technique enabling gene insertion, deletion, and alteration, said Shaoqin Sarah Gong, Vilas distinguished professor in biomedical engineering at the Wisconsin Institute of Discovery, University of Wisconsin–Madison. As part of the Somatic Cell Genome Editing Consortium established last year by the National Institutes of Health (NIH), Gong and colleagues are developing nanoplatforms to deliver Cas9 protein/single guided RNA (sgRNA) ribonucleoprotein complex (RNP) packaged into a nanocapsule. This approach, she said, allows precise control over the ratio of Cas9 and sgRNA within the RNP and enables rapid editing with a low incidence of off-target effects. Like other non-viral vector approaches, it also offers a good safety profile and versatile chemistry, and is easy to scale up, said Gong.

The nanocapsule, composed of a covalently cross-linked yet intracellularly biodegradable polymer coating, has a surface that can be conjugated with a wide array of targeting ligands, said Gong. It is taken up by specifically targeted cells through receptor-mediated endocytosis, she said, and once inside the target cell, the nanocapsule disintegrates and releases the RNP into the cytosol. The RNP is then transported to the nucleus, where it can carry out its editing of the targeted gene, she said. The nanocapsules achieve high editing efficiency even when freeze dried, which provides benefits in terms of purification, long-term storage, transportation, and dosage control, said Gong. She added that the nanocapsule is much less cytotoxic than Lipofectamine, a commercially available reagent often used to deliver DNA or RNA into cells.

Gong and colleagues have tested the efficiency of a nanocapsule targeting the human Alzheimer's precursor protein gene (*APP*) in cell culture, building on the work of her collaborator Subhojit Roy and colleagues, who recently used a CRISPR/Cas9 strategy to selectively silence *APP* through gene editing, suggesting that this may be an effective treatment modality (Sun et al., 2019). Gong and colleagues are also exploring other types of nanoplatforms to target different types of cells and deliver a wide range of hydrophilic payloads, including DNA, mRNA, proteins, and small-molecule drugs.

Novel Delivery Methods

Returning to the challenge of delivery, Junghae Suh, associate professor of bioengineering at Rice University, and Viviana Gradinaru, professor of neuroscience and biological engineering at the California Institute of Technology, addressed from the bioengineering perspective how delivery vectors can be engineered to be more efficient, more specific, and more controllable and how features of gene expression can be controlled.

Gradinaru provided some concrete examples from the field of protein engineering, where directed evolution has emerged as a means to engineer natural products for novel functionality. Working with Frances Arnold, who in 2018 won a Nobel Prize in chemistry (along with co-winners Gregory Winter and George Smith) for her development of the directed evolution approach, Gradinaru and colleagues generated thousands of variants of light-responsive proteins called opsins and then put them through very stringent selection criteria to get opsins that emit light in response to voltage, effectively turning them into voltage sensors (Flytzanis et al., 2014).

The same principles have also been applied to the development of improved viral vectors, said Gradinaru. Using directed evolution, she and her colleagues refined the properties of the AAV9 capsid to enable the virus to cross the blood–brain barrier in rodents, thus creating the PHP.B variant mentioned in Chapter 3 (Chan et al., 2017; Deverman et al., 2016). However, translating this from the rodent to non-human primate brain has proved difficult, in part because of the increased volume of the primate brain and cross-species variations, including different mechanisms to cross the blood–brain barrier, said Gradinaru. It becomes a numbers problem, she said, because meeting these challenges with directed evolution requires the generation of many offspring—as many as 1 billion or more depending on the molecule being targeted. Because no biological screen can fully sample this space, computational biologists, statisticians, and machine learning approaches are essential, she said. The concept is simple, but sounds like magic, she said: You feed training data into the computer, which spits out sequences that can be tested for the presence of desired characteristics.

Gradinaru said that once they had solved the challenge of crossing the blood–brain barrier in rodents, they encountered another challenge that required better opsins. Application of directed evolution and machine learning approaches to this problem yielded improved opsins for systemic delivery, which can be used for minimally invasive optogenetics (Bedbrook et al., in press). Now, in a parallel approach, they are applying directed evolution with deep sequencing to create variants that can achieve biodistribution to specific cell types such as endothelial cells in the vasculature or neurons.

Although the Parkinson's disease (PD) trial failures discussed by Jeffrey Kordower in Chapter 2 may have doomed glial-derived neurotrophic factor and neurturin as treatments for PD, they informed another approach that Kordower and colleagues are now pursuing: using intracellular antibodies (intrabodies) delivered with an AAV vector to clear α-synuclein (Chatterjee et al., 2018). The intrabodies are designed to bind to both monomeric and fibrillar forms of α-synuclein, prevent aggregation, and promote clearance. In a rat model of PD, direct delivery of the AAV-intrabody construct into the substantia nigra has resulted in improved motor behavior and increased intrastriatal dopamine, said Kordower. Next, they are hoping to use better vectors that will enable delivery throughout the brain. Steven Paul, chief executive officer of Karuna Pharmaceuticals, commented that a similar approach has been used to reduce tau pathology in mutant tau transgenic mice, and that this approach seemed to have superior efficacy in reducing tau-dependent neurodegeneration (Liu et al., 2016b).

DIVERSE EXPERTISE NEEDED TO
TACKLE DELIVERY CHALLENGES

Protein engineering and directed evolution have made significant impacts on the development of better vectors to deliver cargo to a specific cell type, said Suh. The next challenge, she said, is to control the level of gene expression in the cargo. Other features of the expression profile that one might want to control include duration, periodicity, and response to the physiological state of the infected cell. To tackle this challenge, Suh advocated enlisting the help of synthetic biologists who apply their expertise in engineering control systems (i.e., inputs and outputs) to solve biological problems. For example, synthetic biologists have developed light-activatable transcriptional activators that optogenetically control gene expression (Olson et al., 2014) (see Figure 6-1). Suh said this group has gone on to demonstrate the multiplex control, that is, the ability to control the expression of two different genes in the same cells.

The next challenge, said Suh, is deciding which genes to deliver for polygenic diseases. Fortunately, she said, systems biologists and computational biologists have already begun applying their expertise to the brain. What they do, she said, is apply data science tools to extract non-obvious patterns from complex datasets so that multipronged therapeutic approaches can be developed to treat complex diseases (Geschwind and Konopka, 2009).

To address the final challenge, administration of gene delivery vectors to the brain and spinal cord, Suh said scientists with expertise in computational fluid dynamics are needed. Through quantitative modeling of the transport of things (e.g., fluids, molecules, proteins, viruses) in complex environments, and applying these models to patient-derived imaging data, these scientists have been able to extract patient-specific three-dimensional maps of the vasculature, understand what blood flow patterns look like in that patient, and provide the information physicians need to decide how to treat the patient. Suh said that we now need to enlist these scientists to develop similar models that can elucidate how things move in and out of the CNS.

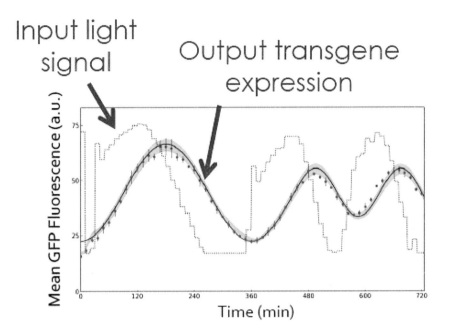

FIGURE 6-1 Optogenetic transcriptional control of gene expression. The input signal (light), represented by the dotted green line, shows the variation in light intensity over time; the corresponding output signal (green fluorescent protein, or GFP, expression) shows the desired sinusoidal oscillations, demonstrating the ability of light to accurately and precisely control gene expression.
SOURCES: Presented by Junghae Suh, April 24, 2019. From Olson et al., 2014.

Suh added that identifying the synthetic biologists, computational biologists, and experts in computational fluid dynamics will not, by itself, be enough. Orchestrating a coherent effort, she said, will require a better structure and more connectors. In an orchestra, she noted, violins sit in one place and cellos in another, with all musical units clearly decoupled from one another. To create a symphony, they must have an organizational structure and a connector (the conductor) that enables them to work together. Similarly, to facilitate the robust solutions and pathways that will move gene therapy for CNS disorders forward, Suh said that connectors are needed who are skilled at forging links between disciplines and mediating effective communication.

Gradinaru added that help from the community and different disciplines would also help evolve vectors to bypass some of the challenges encountered in trying to develop designer AAVs for neuroscience that have the necessary cell type, circuit, organ, and/or region specificity; that can cross the blood–brain barrier or the placenta if intended to be delivered to embryos; and that are capable of carrying large cargo.

Cross-disciplinary collaborations are also needed to translate these new technologies from rodents to non-human primates, said Gradinaru. Because these experiments are difficult and resource intensive, the scientific community has been reluctant to test novel approaches in non-human primates, she said. "You rely on collaborators that are brave enough to test your rodent variants or that are generous enough to give you a few non-human primates to do these assays," said Gradinaru. In an ongoing collaboration with investigators at the NIH/National Institute of Mental Health transgenic marmoset core, she and her colleagues have designed an experiment that tests pooled RNA-barcoded AAV9 variants in the monkeys. Although in its early days, this paradigm has the potential to efficiently, quickly, and cost-effectively screen many capsids in non-human primates, she said.

MOVING BEYOND MONOGENIC DISORDERS

As the examples presented in Chapter 2 illustrate, successful gene-targeted therapies for CNS disorders have thus far been restricted to rare monogenic disorders. However, Chapter 3 described progress in developing gene-targeted therapies for more common and complex polygenic disorders such as PD and Alzheimer's disease (AD) where the neuropathological underpinnings of the disease may not be fully understood. To determine which genes to target, Steven Hyman said there is no shortcut for basic biology. Genetic studies have pointed toward pathways and molecular complexes associated with elevated risk, he said, but to wisely select targets and think about a strategy for target validation one must first fully understand those pathways at a molecular level. Anastasia Khvorova added that translating an understanding of molecular mechanisms into new therapies will also require a clear understanding of how different targets interact with each other.

Developing Gene-Targeted Therapies of Psychiatric and Neurodevelopmental Disorders

Although scientists have begun to tackle complex polygenic disorders with gene therapy, they have not yet begun to apply this therapeutic approach to psychiatric disorders, said Hyman. He asserted that the time has come to think about this challenge while recognizing that clinical applications are a long way off.

Although neuropsychiatric disorders are highly heritable, all common neuropsychiatric disorders are highly polygenic, with phenotypes resulting from myriad small genetic nudges rather than a large genetic shove, said Hyman. He noted that this complicates efforts to identify which genes could be targeted. Moreover, he said, highly penetrant alleles that substantially elevate risk for early-onset behavioral disorders are quickly selected out of the gene pool because these highly disabling illnesses reduce the likelihood that an affected person will have children (Power et al., 2013). Large-effect alleles can occur de novo, but are rarely transmitted, while common and rare variants with low effect sizes can be readily transmitted, said Hyman.

Nonetheless, scientists have created animal models that replicate the human phenotype and have been able to reverse the phenotype by targeting specific genes, suggesting that gene therapy may be feasible. For example, Hyman cited the work of Adrian Bird and colleagues, who were able to reverse neurological defects in a mouse model of Rett syndrome (Guy et al., 2007).

Schizophrenia, however, is far more complex, said Hyman, with hundreds of genome-wide significant loci identified and extreme phenotypic heterogeneity (Huckins et al., 2019). He described a tool that could help scientists roughly stratify affected individuals at a genetic level by creating, for each individual, a weighted sum of risk alleles across the entire genome to produce a polygenic risk score (PRS). The PRS enables stratification of subjects by severity of genetic loading and permits identification of shared common variant risk across phenotypes, said Hyman. It can also help identify important genetic pathways and potentially identify targets for gene therapy interventions, he said. For example, about 70 percent of genome-wide association study (GWAS) hits in AD studies are expressed in microglia and are thought to be involved in inappropriate synapse elimination, said Hyman. He speculated that in schizophrenia, although none of the GWAS hits are expressed in microglia, there may be similar biological processes reached through different pathways such as genes encoding synaptic proteins and complement proteins that signal to microglia, adding that useful target selection can sometimes emerge from analysis of these pathways. What is important, he said, is to understand the biology. Transgenic animal models would require vastly improved methods of multiplexing using gene editing technologies.

The high degree of polygenicity seen in schizophrenia is also seen in common forms of neurodevelopmental disorders such as autism (Gaugler et al., 2014), said Hyman. Indeed, schizophrenia is considered to be neurodevelopmental in origin (Rund, 2018). A recent study by the Autism Sequencing Consortium (ASC) examining 36,000 exomes from affected and unaffected individuals identified 102 genes that are strongly associated with autism, said Joseph Buxbaum, director of the Seaver Autism Center for Research and Treatment at the Icahn School of Medicine at Mount Sinai in New York. Many of the gene mutations that have been identified are highly penetrant with serious deleterious impact and can be parsed into those that are autism specific and less autism specific, Buxbaum said.

Buxbaum summarized data from ASC and the Deciphering Developmental Disorders Study in the United Kingdom, which sequenced the genomes and phenotyped more than 4,000 individuals with severe developmental disorders (Deciphering Developmental Disorders Study, 2015). Together, he said, these studies and others have implicated multiple pathways. The genes discovered to date are overwhelmingly contributing to dominant disorders. The importance of a dominant disorder, said Buxbaum, is that there is a second allele that can be manipulated. He said most mutations identified to date result in a loss of function and are dose sensitive, typically displaying a U-shaped curve indicating that problems arise when there is either too much or too little gene expression. Most of the mutations result in severe conditions, he said, and in some cases re-expression of the gene later in life can be beneficial. For example, Guoping Feng and colleagues reported that in mouse models, mutations in *SHANK3* result in synaptic dysfunction and autistic-like behaviors, but that re-expressing the gene in adult mice improved neural function and behavior, said Buxbaum (Mei et al., 2016).

Among the genes identified in these studies, those with the strongest findings are relatively common and highly penetrant, said Buxbaum. For example, *SHANK3* haploinsufficiency explains about 0.5 percent of autism cases and 0.5 percent of intellectual disability cases, according to some studies (Betancur and Buxbaum, 2013), while other studies suggest an even higher association of *SHANK3* with autism, he said. Loss of *SHANK3* is called Phelan-McDermid syndrome (PMS), said Buxbaum. Taking PMS as one example, Buxbaum made the following points. Given that genetic testing can readily identify PMS; that it is thought to be fully penetrant with many potential biomarkers, rodent models, and even a primate model; and that there is an effective and engaged family foundation, Buxbaum suggested that this disorder may be an excellent target for gene therapy. Moreover, he said, a successful gene therapy for PMS might be repositioned to treat other forms of autism where there is no *SHANK3* mutation, but where overlapping pathways are disrupted via other mechanisms. This is but one example, he said, suggesting there are already several dozen other known genes that are natural targets for gene therapy.

TARGETING NON-CODING RNAs

While most of the workshop discussions focused on genes that encode proteins, as much as 90 percent of genetic variants detected in GWAS are for non-coding genes, said Hyman. Only about one-third of those are known to be mapped to a particular gene, and even for those the directionality of their effect is mostly unknown, he said. But the fine mapping that is being achieved now may provide much of that information. Beverly

Davidson challenged workshop participants to think about how these non-coding RNAs might be targeted, how target engagement might be assessed, and efficacy might be measured.

Khvorova suggested that non-coding RNA is as targetable as coding RNA. Modeling the expression of any of these genes can be accomplished with a panel of tools (e.g., animal models), she said, even when the mechanisms are unclear, she said. Hyman added that the non-coding portion of the genome may be the most evolvable and thus important in the context of developing gene-targeted therapies. Induced pluripotent stem cells, organoids, and xenotransplanted human neurons are increasingly being used in these studies, he said. Bhattarcharyya suggested that regulation of splicing may be particularly useful for targeting non-coding RNAs.

Abeliovich added that our growing knowledge of endogenous regulatory mechanisms may be leveraged in the development of gene therapeutics. For example, he said, a few examples of single-nucleotide polymorphisms appear to be regulatory and potentially disease modifying. A complicating issue, said Khvorova, is that many non-coding RNAs are only expressed in early developmental stages and not expressed or expressed at different levels or in different combinations in adults, adding complexity to data interpretation.

Sarah DeVos added that cells may also produce naturally occurring self-regulatory antisense that could potentially be targeted. Davidson said this is being attempted in some neonatal epilepsies caused by haploinsufficiency, which potentially could be blocked by targeting non-coding RNA that modulates that transcript.

POTENTIAL FOR PRE-COMPETITIVE COLLABORATION

Henderson commented that, while it is important that each company create its own intellectual property around specific programs, the large number of variables associated with gene-targeted therapies remains a significant challenge for individual companies. He suggested exploring the potential of pre-competitive partnerships to establish reproducible baseline data for standardized preparations of widely used capsids in primate models, including routes of administration and safety issues. He further suggested that although treating the adult brain will be "the next frontier," this presents additional challenges not encountered in trials that enrolled infants and children. Ronald Crystal added standardizing assays for vectors to the list of issues that might be best addressed by pre-competitive partnerships. Hao Wang, global program leader for the CNS therapeutic area at Takeda Pharmaceuticals, noted that immune-related issues could also fall into potential collaborative activities.

Investing in Natural History Studies

To reach more diseases, particularly rare and ultrarare diseases, a collaborative platform approach starting with a natural history cohort is critical, added Petra Kaufmann. Such an approach could allow for the application of advanced and novel technologies and other resources to rare populations and provide recruitment registries and control populations, she said. Holly Tabor added that engaging with patients and patient communities can enable the building of natural history study databases. Rare disease groups and patients have long advocated for paying more attention to the natural history of their disorders, she said. Story Landis noted that academic groups and patient groups may not be aware of what is needed to make a natural history study useful for those who are conducting clinical trials.

Natural history studies are essential to developing compelling clinical trials, said Landis. Many single-gene defects are ripe for therapy development, she said, but in the absence of the natural history, selecting appropriate endpoints is not possible. Kaufmann agreed, noting that natural history studies should include "regulatory actionable" outcome measures. Kathleen Reape also noted that in ultrarare diseases, natural history data may be used as the control data. Indeed, in Chapter 2, Kaufmann described how natural history data were used in this way in the AVXS-101 trial, which led to the approval of a gene replacement therapy for SMA.

Landis said the National Institute of Neurological Disorders and Stroke (NINDS) has a clinical readiness funding program to support partnerships between academics and patient groups for natural history studies and identification of clinical endpoints. Walter Koroshetz, director of NINDS, reiterated Landis's comment, noting that NIH has funded several programs relevant to these proceedings, including not only natural history studies for nine different diseases, but other programs for biomarker validation and clinical trial readiness as well. They are also funding industry and disease collaborations to conduct clinical trials, he said. Frank Bennett added that having industry participation in the design of natural history studies is critical.

FINAL REMARKS

Treating CNS disorders by gene modification has become a reality in clinical applications, Shihabuddin said in her workshop wrap-up remarks. Moreover, the powerful platforms that have led to successful development of gene-targeted therapies for rare diseases have the potential to be tailored to target more common disorders, she said. Shihabuddin noted the many technical challenges that remain, including optimizing more efficient delivery to the correct brain regions and cell types, increasing the potency of antisense oligonucleotides and RNA interference chemistries, and designing bridging studies to accelerate moving from first generation to safer and more potent second generation vectors and other products.

Innovations in these and other areas may help to increase the efficacy of treatments and applicability to a broader range of diseases and may also drive down costs and improve patient access to treatments, said Shihabuddin. To address the challenges faced, she called for collaboration across academics, industry, NIH, regulators, and patient advocacy groups.

Appendix A

References

Abeliovich, A., and A. D. Gitler. 2016. Defects in trafficking bridge Parkinson's disease pathology and genetics. *Nature* 539(7628):207–216.

Adams, D., A. Gonzalez-Duarte, W. D. O'Riordan, C. C. Yang, M. Ueda, A. V. Kristen, I. Tournev, H. H. Schmidt, T. Coelho, J. L. Berk, K. P. Lin, G. Vita, S. Attarian, V. Plante-Bordeneuve, M. M. Mezei, J. M. Campistol, J. Buades, T. H. Brannagan, 3rd, B. J. Kim, J. Oh, Y. Parman, Y. Sekijima, P. N. Hawkins, S. D. Solomon, M. Polydefkis, P. J. Dyck, P. J. Gandhi, S. Goyal, J. Chen, A. L. Strahs, S. V. Nochur, M. T. Sweetser, P. P. Garg, A. K. Vaishnaw, J. A. Gollob, and O. B. Suhr. 2018. Patisiran, an RNAi therapeutic, for hereditary transthyretin amyloidosis. *New England Journal of Medicine* 379(1):11–21.

Amado, D. A., J. M. Rieders, F. Diatta, P. Hernandez-Con, A. Singer, J. T. Mak, J. Zhang, E. Lancaster, B. L. Davidson, and A. S. Chen-Plotkin. 2019. AAV-mediated progranulin delivery to a mouse model of progranulin deficiency causes T cell-mediated toxicity. *Molecular Therapy* 27(2):465–478.

Banez-Coronel, M., F. Ayhan, A. D. Tarabochia, T. Zu, B. A. Perez, S. K. Tusi, O. Pletnikova, D. R. Borchelt, C. A. Ross, R. L. Margolis, A. T. Yachnis, J. C. Troncoso, and L. P. Ranum. 2015. RAN translation in Huntington disease. *Neuron* 88(4):667–677.

Bedbrook, C. N., K. K. Yang, J. E. Robinson, V. Gradinaru, and F. H. Arnold. In press. Machine learning-guided channelrhodopsin engineering enables minimally-invasive optogenetics. *Nature Methods*.

Bennett, J., M. Ashtari, J. Wellman, K. A. Marshall, L. L. Cyckowski, D. C. Chung, S. McCague, E. A. Pierce, Y. Chen, J. L. Bennicelli, X. Zhu, G. S. Ying, J. Sun, J. F. Wright, A. Auricchio, F. Simonelli, K. S. Shindler, F. Mingozzi, K. A. High, and A. M. Maguire. 2012. AAV2 gene therapy readministration in three adults with congenital blindness. *Science Translational Medicine* 4(120):120ra115.

Bennicelli, J., J. F. Wright, A. Komaromy, J. B. Jacobs, B. Hauck, O. Zelenaia, F. Mingozzi, D. Hui, D. Chung, T. S. Rex, Z. Wei, G. Qu, S. Zhou, C. Zeiss, V. R. Arruda, G. M. Acland, L. F. Dell'Osso, K. A. High, A. M. Maguire, and J. Bennett. 2008. Reversal of blindness in animal models of leber congenital amaurosis using optimized AAV2-mediated gene transfer. *Molecular Therapy* 16(3):458–465.

Betancur, C., and J. D. Buxbaum. 2013. SHANK3 haploinsufficiency: A "common" but under-diagnosed highly penetrant monogenic cause of autism spectrum disorders. *Molecular Autism* 4(1):17.

Bevan, A. K., S. Duque, K. D. Foust, P. R. Morales, L. Braun, L. Schmelzer, C. M. Chan, M. McCrate, L. G. Chicoine, B. D. Coley, P. N. Porensky, S. J. Kolb, J. R. Mendell, A. H. Burghes, and B. K. Kaspar. 2011. Systemic gene delivery in large species for targeting spinal cord, brain, and peripheral tissues for pediatric disorders. *Molecular Therapy* 19(11):1971–1980.

Buchman, A. S., L. Yu, R. S. Wilson, S. E. Leurgans, S. Nag, J. M. Shulman, L. L. Barnes, J. A. Schneider, and D. A. Bennett. 2019. Progressive Parkinsonism in older adults is related to the burden of mixed brain pathologies. *Neurology* 92(16):e1821–e1830.

Challis, R. C., S. R. Kumar, K. Y. Chan, C. Challis, K. Beadle, M. J. Jang, H. M. Kim, P. S. Rajendran, J. D. Tompkins, K. Shivkumar, B. E. Deverman, and V. Gradinaru. 2019. Systemic AAV vectors for widespread and targeted gene delivery in rodents. *Nature Protocols* 14:379–414.

Chan, K. Y., M. J. Jang, B. B. Yoo, A. Greenbaum, N. Ravi, W. L. Wu, L. Sanchez-Guardado, C. Lois, S. K. Mazmanian, B. E. Deverman, and V. Gradinaru. 2017. Engineered AAVs for efficient noninvasive gene delivery to the central and peripheral nervous systems. *Nature Neuroscience* 20(8):1172–1179.

Chatterjee, D., M. Bhatt, D. Butler, E. De Genst, C. M. Dobson, A. Messer, and J. H. Kordower. 2018. Proteasome-targeted nanobodies alleviate pathology and functional decline in an alpha-synuclein-based Parkinson's disease model. *npj Parkinson's Disease* 4:25.

Christopher, P. P., P. S. Appelbaum, D. Truong, K. Albert, L. Maranda, and C. Lidz. 2017. Reducing therapeutic misconception: A randomized intervention trial in hypothetical clinical trials. *PLoS ONE* 12(9):e0184224.

Chu, Y., A. S. Buchman, C. W. Olanow, and J. H. Kordower. 2018. Do subjects with minimal motor features have prodromal Parkinson disease? *Annals of Neurology* 83(3):562–574.

Chung, D. C., S. McCague, Z. F. Yu, S. Thill, J. DiStefano-Pappas, J. Bennett, D. Cross, K. Marshall, J. Wellman, and K. A. High. 2018. Novel mobility test to assess functional vision in patients with inherited retinal dystrophies. *Clinical & Experimental Ophthalmology* 46(3):247–259.

Dahl, M., A. Doyle, K. Olsson, J. E. Mansson, A. R. A. Marques, M. Mirzaian, J. M. Aerts, M. Ehinger, M. Rothe, U. Modlich, A. Schambach, and S. Karlsson. 2015. Lentiviral gene therapy using cellular promoters cures Type 1 Gaucher disease in mice. *Molecular Therapy* 23(5):835–844.

Deciphering Developmental Disorders Study. 2015. Large-scale discovery of novel genetic causes of developmental disorders. *Nature* 519(7542):223–228.

Deverman, B. E., P. L. Pravdo, B. P. Simpson, S. R. Kumar, K. Y. Chan, A. Banerjee, W. L. Wu, B. Yang, N. Huber, S. P. Pasca, and V. Gradinaru. 2016. Cre-dependent selection yields AAV variants for widespread gene transfer to the adult brain. *Nature Biotechnology* 34(2):204–209.

DeVos, S. L., R. L. Miller, K. M. Schoch, B. B. Holmes, C. S. Kebodeaux, A. J. Wegener, G. Chen, T. Shen, H. Tran, B. Nichols, T. A. Zanardi, H. B. Kordasiewicz, E. E. Swayze, C. F. Bennett, M. I. Diamond, and T. M. Miller. 2017. Tau reduction prevents neuronal loss and reverses pathological tau deposition and seeding in mice with tauopathy. *Science Translational Medicine* 9(374):eaag0481.

Duque, S. I., W. D. Arnold, P. Odermatt, X. Li, P. N. Porensky, L. Schmelzer, K. Meyer, S. J. Kolb, D. Schumperli, B. K. Kaspar, and A. H. Burghes. 2015. A large animal model of spinal muscular atrophy and correction of phenotype. *Annals of Neurology* 77(3):399–414.

Farrar, M. A., and M. C. Kiernan. 2015. The genetics of spinal muscular atrophy: Progress and challenges. *Neurotherapeutics* 12(2):290–302.

FDA (Food and Drug Administration). 2019. *May 24, 2019 approval letter—zolgensmsa.* https://www.fda.gov/media/126130/download (accessed May 25, 2019).

Finkel, R. S., M. P. McDermott, P. Kaufmann, B. T. Darras, W. K. Chung, D. M. Sproule, P. B. Kang, A. R. Foley, M. L. Yang, W. B. Martens, M. Oskoui, A. M. Glanzman, J. Flickinger, J. Montes, S. Dunaway, J. O'Hagen, J. Quigley, S. Riley, M. Benton, P. A. Ryan, M. Montgomery, J. Marra, C. Gooch, and D. C. De Vivo. 2014. Observational study of spinal muscular atrophy type I and implications for clinical trials. *Neurology* 83(9):810–817.

Finkel, R. S., C. A. Chiriboga, J. Vajsar, J. W. Day, J. Montes, D. C. De Vivo, M. Yamashita, F. Rigo, G. Hung, E. Schneider, D. A. Norris, S. Xia, C. F. Bennett, and K. M. Bishop. 2016. Treatment of infantile-onset spinal muscular atrophy with nusinersen: A phase 2, open-label, dose-escalation study. *The Lancet* 388(10063):3017–3026.

Finkel, R. S., E. Mercuri, B. T. Darras, A. M. Connolly, N. L. Kuntz, J. Kirschner, C. A. Chiriboga, K. Saito, L. Servais, E. Tizzano, H. Topaloglu, M. Tulinius, J. Montes, A. M. Glanzman, K. Bishop, Z. J. Zhong, S. Gheuens, C. F. Bennett, E. Schneider, W. Farwell, D. C. De Vivo, and E. S. Group. 2017. Nusinersen versus sham control in infantile-onset spinal muscular atrophy. *New England Journal of Medicine* 377(18):1723–1732.

Flytzanis, N. C., C. N. Bedbrook, H. Chiu, M. K. Engqvist, C. Xiao, K. Y. Chan, P. W. Sternberg, F. H. Arnold, and V. Gradinaru. 2014. Archaerhodopsin variants with enhanced voltage-sensitive fluorescence in mammalian and Caenorhabditis elegans neurons. *Nature Communications* 5:4894.

Foust, K. D., X. Wang, V. L. McGovern, L. Braun, A. K. Bevan, A. M. Haidet, T. T. Le, P. R. Morales, M. M. Rich, A. H. Burghes, and B. K. Kaspar. 2010. Rescue of the spinal muscular atrophy phenotype in a mouse model by early postnatal delivery of SMN. *Nature Biotechnology* 28(3):271–274.

Gao, F. B., and J. D. Richter. 2017. Microsatellite expansion diseases: Repeat toxicity found in translation. *Neuron* 93(2):249–251.

Garrison, L. P., T. Jackson, D. Paul, and M. Kenston. 2019. Value-based pricing for emerging gene therapies: The economic case for a higher cost-effectiveness threshold. *Journal of Managed Care & Specialty Pharmacy* 25(7):793–799.

Gaugler, T., L. Klei, S. J. Sanders, C. A. Bodea, A. P. Goldberg, A. B. Lee, M. Mahajan, D. Manaa, Y. Pawitan, J. Reichert, S. Ripke, S. Sandin, P. Sklar, O. Svantesson, A. Reichenberg, C. M. Hultman, B. Devlin, K. Roeder, and J. D. Buxbaum. 2014. Most genetic risk for autism resides with common variation. *Nature Genetics* 46(8):881–885.

Geschwind, D. H., and G. Konopka. 2009. Neuroscience in the era of functional genomics and systems biology. *Nature* 461(7266):908–915.

Gray, S. J., B. L. Blake, H. E. Criswell, S. C. Nicolson, R. J. Samulski, T. J. McCown, and W. Li. 2010. Directed evolution of a novel adeno-associated virus (AAV) vector that crosses the seizure-compromised blood–brain barrier (BBB). *Molecular Therapy* 18(3):570–578.

Guy, J., J. Gan, J. Selfridge, S. Cobb, and A. Bird. 2007. Reversal of neurological defects in a mouse model of Rett Syndrome. *Science* 315(5815):1143–1147.

Henderson, G. E., L. R. Churchill, A. M. Davis, M. M. Easter, C. Grady, S. Joffe, N. Kass, N. M. P. King, C. W. Lidz, F. G. Miller, D. K. Nelson, J. Peppercorn, B. B. Rothschild, P. Sankar, B. S. Wilfond, and C. R. Zimmer. 2007. Clinical trials and medical care: Defining the therapeutic misconception. *PLoS Medicine* 4(11):e324.

Hua, Y., K. Sahashi, G. Hung, F. Rigo, M. A. Passini, C. F. Bennett, and A. R. Krainer. 2010. Antisense correction of SMN2 splicing in the CNS rescues necrosis in a type III SMA mouse model. *Genes & Development* 24(15):1634–1644.

Huckins, L. M., A. Dobbyn, D. M. Ruderfer, G. Hoffman, W. Wang, A. F. Pardinas, V. M. Rajagopal, T. D. Als, H. T. Nguyen, K. Girdhar, J. Boocock, P. Roussos, M. Fromer, R. Kramer, E. Domenici, E. R. Gamazon, S. Purcell, CommonMind Consortium, The Schizophrenia Working Group of the Psychiatric Genomics Consortium, iPSYCH-GEMS Schizophrenia Working Group, D. Demontis, A. D. Borglum, J. T. R. Walters, M. C. O'Donovan, P. Sullivan, M. J. Owen, B. Devlin, S. K. Sieberts, N. J. Cox, H. K. Im, P. Sklar, and E. A. Stahl. 2019. Gene expression imputation across multiple brain regions provides insights into schizophrenia risk. *Nature Genetics* 51(4):659–674.

ICER (Institute for Clinical and Economic Review). 2019. *Spinraza and zolgensma for spinal muscular atrophy: Effectiveness and value: Final evidence report*. https://icer-review.org/wp-content/uploads/2018/07/ICER_SMA_Final_Evidence_Report_040319.pdf (accessed August 9, 2019).

Jonsen, A. R. 2007. The god squad and the origins of transplantation ethics and policy. *The Journal of Law, Medicine & Ethics* 35(2):238–240.

Kaltenboeck, A., and P. B. Bach. 2018. Value-based pricing for drugs: Theme and variations. *JAMA* 319(21):2165–2166.

Kaufmann, P., M. P. McDermott, B. T. Darras, R. S. Finkel, D. M. Sproule, P. B. Kang, M. Oskoui, A. Constantinescu, C. L. Gooch, A. R. Foley, M. L. Yang, R. Tawil, W. K. Chung, W. B. Martens, J. Montes, V. Battista, J. O'Hagen, S. Dunaway, J. Flickinger, J. Quigley, S. Riley, A. M. Glanzman, M. Benton, P. A. Ryan, M. Punyanitya, M. J. Montgomery, J. Marra, B. Koo, D. C. De Vivo, Muscle Study Group, and Pediatric Neuromuscular Clinical Research Network for Spinal Muscular Atrophy. 2012. Prospective cohort study of spinal muscular atrophy types 2 and 3. *Neurology* 79(18):1889–1897.

Khvorova, A., and J. K. Watts. 2017. The chemical evolution of oligonucleotide therapies of clinical utility. *Nature Biotechnology* 35(3):238–248.

Kolb, S. J., C. S. Coffey, J. W. Yankey, K. Krosschell, W. D. Arnold, S. B. Rutkove, K. J. Swoboda, S. P. Reyna, A. Sakonju, B. T. Darras, R. Shell, N. Kuntz, D. Castro, J. Parsons, A. M. Connolly, C. A. Chiriboga, C. McDonald, W. B. Burnette, K. Werner, M. Thangarajh, P. B. Shieh, E. Finanger, M. E. Cudkowicz, M. M. McGovern, D. E. McNeil, R. Finkel, S. T. Iannaccone, E. Kaye, A. Kingsley, S. R. Renusch, V. L. McGovern, X. Wang, P. G. Zaworski, T. W. Prior, A. H. M. Burghes, A. Bartlett, J. T. Kissel, and NeuroNEXT Clinical Trial Network on behalf of the NN101 SMA Biomarker Investigators. 2017. Natural history of infantile-onset spinal muscular atrophy. *Annals of Neurology* 82(6):883–891.

Kole, R., and A. M. Krieg. 2015. Exon skipping therapy for Duchenne muscular dystrophy. *Advanced Drug Delivery Reviews* 87:104–107.

Kordower, J. H., S. Palfi, E. Y. Chen, S. Y. Ma, T. Sendera, E. J. Cochran, E. J. Mufson, R. Penn, C. G. Goetz, and C. D. Comella. 1999. Clinicopathological findings following intraventricular glial-derived neurotrophic factor treatment in a patient with Parkinson's disease. *Annals of Neurology* 46(3):419–424.

Kordower, J. H., M. E. Emborg, J. Bloch, S. Y. Ma, Y. Chu, L. Leventhal, J. McBride, E. Y. Chen, S. Palfi, B. Z. Roitberg, W. D. Brown, J. E. Holden, R. Pyzalski, M. D. Taylor, P. Carvey, Z. Ling, D. Trono, P. Hantraye, N. Deglon, and P. Aebischer. 2000. Neurodegeneration prevented by lentiviral vector delivery of GDNF in primate models of Parkinson's disease. *Science* 290(5492):767–773.

Kornegay, J. N. 2017. The golden retriever model of Duchenne muscular dystrophy. *Skeletal Muscle* 7(1):9.

Li, L., E. K. Dimitriadis, Y. Yang, J. Li, Z. Yuan, C. Qiao, C. Beley, R. H. Smith, L. Garcia, and R. M. Kotin. 2013. Production and characterization of novel recombinant adeno-associated virus replicative-form genomes: A eukaryotic source of DNA for gene transfer. *PLoS ONE* 8(8):e69879.

Liu, G., B. Boot, J. J. Locascio, I. E. Jansen, S. Winder-Rhodes, S. Eberly, A. Elbaz, A. Brice, B. Ravina, J. J. van Hilten, F. Cormier-Dequaire, J. C. Corvol, R. A. Barker, P. Heutink, J. Marinus, C. H. Williams-Gray, C. R. Scherzer, and International Genetics of Parkinson Disease Progression Consortium. 2016a. Specifically neuropathic Gaucher's mutations accelerate cognitive decline in Parkinson's. *Annals of Neurology* 80(5):674–685.

Liu, W., L. Zhao, B. Blackman, M. Parmar, M. Y. Wong, T. Woo, F. Yu, M. J. Chiuchiolo, D. Sondhi, S. M. Kaminsky, R. G. Crystal, and S. M. Paul. 2016b. Vectored intracerebral immunization with the anti-tau monoclonal antibody PHF1 markedly reduces tau pathology in mutant tau transgenic mice. *Journal of Neuroscience* 36(49):12425–12435.

Lo Bianco, C., N. Deglon, W. Pralong, and P. Aebischer. 2004. Lentiviral nigral delivery of GDNF does not prevent neurodegeneration in a genetic rat model of Parkinson's disease. *Neurobiology of Disease* 17(2):283–289.

Lundstrom, K. 2018. Viral vectors in gene therapy. *Diseases* 6(2):42.

Mei, Y., P. Monteiro, Y. Zhou, J. A. Kim, X. Gao, Z. Fu, and G. Feng. 2016. Adult restoration of Shank3 expression rescues selective autistic-like phenotypes. *Nature* 530(7591):481–484.

Mendell, J. R., S. Al-Zaidy, R. Shell, W. D. Arnold, L. R. Rodino-Klapac, T. W. Prior, L. Lowes, L. Alfano, K. Berry, K. Church, J. T. Kissel, S. Nagendran, J. L'Italien, D. M. Sproule, C. Wells, J. A. Cardenas, M. D. Heitzer, A. Kaspar, S. Corcoran, L. Braun, S. Likhite, C. Miranda, K. Meyer, K. D. Foust, A. H. M. Burghes, and B. K. Kaspar. 2017. Single-dose gene-replacement therapy for spinal muscular atrophy. *New England Journal of Medicine* 377(18):1713–1722.

Mintrom, M., and R. Bollard. 2009. Governing controversial science: Lessons from stem cell research. *Policy and Society* 28(4):301–314.

Monteys, A. M., S. A. Ebanks, M. S. Keiser, and B. L. Davidson. 2017. CRISPR/Cas9 editing of the mutant Huntingtin allele in vitro and in vivo. *Molecular Therapy* 25(1):12–23.

Morabito, G., S. G. Giannelli, G. Ordazzo, S. Bido, V. Castoldi, M. Indrigo, T. Cabassi, S. Cattaneo, M. Luoni, C. Cancellieri, A. Sessa, M. Bacigaluppi, S. Taverna, L. Leocani, J. L. Lanciego, and V. Broccoli. 2017. AAV-PHP.B-mediated global-scale expression in the mouse nervous system enables GBA1 gene therapy for wide protection from synucleinopathy. *Molecular Therapy* 25(12):2727–2742.

Olson, E. J., L. A. Hartsough, B. P. Landry, R. Shroff, and J. J. Tabor. 2014. Characterizing bacterial gene circuit dynamics with optically programmed gene expression signals. *Nature Methods* 11(4):449–455.

Pacione, M., C. E. Siskind, J. W. Day, and H. K. Tabor. 2019. Perspectives on Spinraza (nusinersen) treatment study: Views of individuals and parents of children diagnosed with spinal muscular atrophy. *Journal of Neuromuscular Diseases* 6(1):119–131.

Palfi, S., J. M. Gurruchaga, H. Lepetit, K. Howard, G. S. Ralph, S. Mason, G. Gouello, P. Domenech, P. C. Buttery, P. Hantraye, N. J. Tuckwell, R. A. Barker, and K. A. Mitrophanous. 2018. Long-term follow-up of a phase I/II study of prosavin, a lentiviral vector gene therapy for Parkinson's disease. *Human Gene Therapy Clinical Development* 29(3):148–155.

Paton, D. M. 2017. Nusinersen: Antisense oligonucleotide to increase SMN protein production in spinal muscular atrophy. *Drugs of Today (Barcelona, Spain: 1998)* 53(6):327–337.

Power, R. A., S. Kyaga, R. Uher, J. H. MacCabe, N. Langstrom, M. Landen, P. McGuffin, C. M. Lewis, P. Lichtenstein, and A. C. Svensson. 2013. Fecundity of patients with schizophrenia, autism, bipolar disorder, depression, anorexia nervosa, or substance abuse vs their unaffected siblings. *JAMA Psychiatry* 70(1):22–30.

Rayaprolu, V., S. Kruse, R. Kant, B. Venkatakrishnan, N. Movahed, D. Brooke, B. Lins, A. Bennett, T. Potter, R. McKenna, M. Agbandje-McKenna, and B. Bothner. 2013. Comparative analysis of adeno-associated virus capsid stability and dynamics. *Journal of Virology* 87(24):13150–13160.

Rudnik-Schoneborn, S., C. Berg, K. Zerres, C. Betzler, T. Grimm, T. Eggermann, K. Eggermann, R. Wirth, B. Wirth, and R. Heller. 2009. Genotype–phenotype studies in infantile spinal muscular atrophy (SMA) type I in Germany: Implications for clinical trials and genetic counselling. *Clinical Genetics* 76(2):168–178.

Rund, B. R. 2018. The research evidence for schizophrenia as a neurodevelopmental disorder. *Scandinavian Journal of Psychology* 59(1):49–58.

Russell, S., J. Bennett, J. A. Wellman, D. C. Chung, Z. F. Yu, A. Tillman, J. Wittes, J. Pappas, O. Elci, S. McCague, D. Cross, K. A. Marshall, J. Walshire, T. L. Kehoe, H. Reichert, M. Davis, L. Raffini, L. A. George, F. P. Hudson, L. Dingfield, X. Zhu, J. A. Haller, E. H. Sohn, V. B. Mahajan, W. Pfeifer, M. Weckmann, C. Johnson, D. Gewaily, A. Drack, E. Stone, K. Wachtel, F. Simonelli, B. P. Leroy, J. F. Wright, K. A. High, and A. M. Maguire. 2017a. Efficacy and safety of voretigene neparvovec (AAV2-hRPE65v2) in patients with RPE65-mediated inherited retinal dystrophy: A randomised, controlled, open-label, phase 3 trial. *The Lancet* 390(10097):849–860.

Russell, S. R., J. Bennett, J. A. Wellman, D. C. Chung, K. A. High, Z. Yu, A. Tillman, and A. M. Maguire. 2017b. Year 2 results for a phase 3 trial of voretigene neparvovec in biallelic *RPE65*-mediated inherited retinal disease. Poster presented at the Association for Research in Vision and Ophthalmology Annual Meeting, May 7–11, 2017, Baltimore, MD.

Sardi, S. P., J. Clarke, C. Viel, M. Chan, T. J. Tamsett, C. M. Treleaven, J. Bu, L. Sweet, M. A. Passini, J. C. Dodge, W. H. Yu, R. L. Sidman, S. H. Cheng, and L. S. Shihabuddin. 2013. Augmenting CNS glucocerebrosidase activity as a therapeutic strategy for Parkinsonism and other Gaucher-related synucleinopathies. *Proceedings of the National Academy of Sciences of the United States of America* 110(9):3537–3542.

Sathasivam, K., A. Neueder, T. A. Gipson, C. Landles, A. C. Benjamin, M. K. Bondulich, D. L. Smith, R. L. Faull, R. A. Roos, D. Howland, P. J. Detloff, D. E. Housman, and G. P. Bates. 2013. Aberrant splicing of HTT generates the pathogenic exon 1 protein in Huntington disease. *Proceedings of the National Academy of Sciences of the United States of America* 110(6):2366–2370.

Sibbald, B. 2001. Death but one unintended consequence of gene-therapy trial. *CMAJ* 164(11):1612.

Sidransky, E., T. Samaddar, and N. Tayebi. 2009. Mutations in GBA are associated with familial Parkinson disease susceptibility and age at onset. *Neurology* 73(17):1424–1425, author reply 1425–1426.

Steinbrook, R. 2008. The Gelsinger case. In *The Oxford textbook of clinical research ethics*, edited by E. J. Emanuel, C. G. Grady, R. A. Crouch, R. K. Lie, F. G. Miller, and D. D. Wendler. New York: Oxford University Press. Pp. 110–120.

Sun, J., J. Carlson-Stevermer, U. Das, M. Shen, M. Delenclos, A. M. Snead, S. Y. Koo, L. Wang, D. Qiao, J. Loi, A. J. Petersen, M. Stockton, A. Bhattacharyya, M. V. Jones, X. Zhao, P. J. McLean, A. A. Sproul, K. Saha, and S. Roy. 2019. CRISPR/Cas9 editing of APP C-terminus attenuates beta-cleavage and promotes alpha-cleavage. *Nature Communications* 10(1):53.

Appendix B

Workshop Agenda

Advancing Gene-Targeted Therapies for
Central Nervous System Disorders: A Workshop

April 23–24, 2019
National Academy of Sciences Building
2101 Constitution Avenue, NW
Washington, DC

Background:

This public workshop will bring together experts and key stakeholders from academia, government, industry, and nonprofit organizations to explore approaches for advancing the development of gene-targeted therapies for central nervous system (CNS) disorders, including approaches that target nucleic acids, such as adeno-associated viruses (AAVs), antisense oligonucleotides (ASOs), and RNA interference, as well as gene product-targeted therapies.

Workshop Objectives:

Invited presentations and discussions will be designed to:

- Provide an overview of the current landscape of gene-targeted therapy approaches for CNS disorders.

- Discuss lessons learned from recent advances in gene therapy and ASO development for retinal dystrophy and spinal muscular atrophy (SMA).
- Compare features of different gene-targeted therapy approaches in development for CNS disorders, and discuss approaches to matching the approach to specific diseases; addressing their respective administration, distribution, and dose challenges; and exploring potential long-term effects.
- Explore clinical development—including biomarker and clinical endpoint selection, trial design to demonstrate disease modification, and the regulatory path—for gene-targeted therapy approaches for rare genetic disorders that have more variable onset and slower progression.
- Discuss what it would take to move beyond rare genetic disorders to develop gene-targeted therapy approaches for more common, heterogeneous disorders such as Alzheimer's and Parkinson's diseases.
- Explore opportunities for catalyzing development of gene-targeted therapy approaches for nervous system disorders, including potential collaborative efforts among sectors and across disorders.

April 23, 2019

1:30 p.m.   Welcome and Overview of Workshop
STORY LANDIS, Co-Chair, Forum on Neuroscience and Nervous System Disorders (*Co-Chair*)
LAMYA SHIHABUDDIN, Sanofi (*Co-Chair*)

SESSION I: CURRENT LANDSCAPE AND LESSONS LEARNED

Objectives:

- Provide an overview of the current landscape of gene-targeted therapy approaches for central nervous system disorders.
- Explore lessons learned from gene and ASO therapies that have achieved Food and Drug Administration approval—including translation plans and which animal models were used in preclinical studies, use of dog models for *RPE65*, role of natural history studies for SMA therapy, and other lessons learned in translation to clinical development.

- Examine lessons learned from gene therapy efforts that were not successful, including neurotrophins for neurodegenerative diseases.

1:40 p.m. Session Overview
LAMYA SHIHABUDDIN, Sanofi (*Moderator*)

1:45 p.m. RPE65 Gene Therapy
KATHLEEN REAPE, Spark Therapeutics

2:00 p.m. ASO Therapy for SMA
C. FRANK BENNETT, Ionis

2:15 p.m. Gene Therapy for SMA
PETRA KAUFMANN, AveXis

2:30 p.m. Lessons Learned from Unsuccessful Gene Therapy Trials of Neurotrophins for Neurodegenerative Diseases
JEFFREY KORDOWER, Rush University

2:45 p.m. Panel Discussion: Preclinical Studies, Delivery Methods, and Clinical Trial Issues Focused on These Cases with the Intent to Identify General Issues That Will and Will Not Apply to Other Applications/Diseases
The speakers above will be joined by panelists:
RONALD CRYSTAL, Weill Cornell Medicine
CHRISTOPHER HENDERSON, Biogen

3:25 p.m. General Discussion

3:45 p.m. BREAK

SESSION II: SELECTING GENE-TARGETED THERAPY APPROACHES FOR CNS DISORDERS

Objectives:

- Discuss the promise and potential pitfalls of gene-targeted therapies specifically for CNS disorders.
- For CNS disorders, compare features of different therapies that target nucleic acid, including AAVs, ASOs, and RNA interference, as well as gene product–targeted therapies.

- Explore what makes a CNS disorder potentially amenable to treatment via gene-targeted therapies and how to match therapy modality and mechanism of action to specific diseases.
- Discuss when uncontrolled overexpression is appropriate.

4:00 p.m.   Session Overview
             BEVERLY DAVIDSON, Children's Hospital of Philadelphia
             and University of Pennsylvania School of Medicine
             (*Moderator*)

4:05 p.m.   Speakers
             ANASTASIA KHVOROVA, University of Massachusetts
             Medical School
             ASA ABELIOVICH, Prevail Therapeutics
             SARAH DEVOS, Denali Therapeutics

4:35 p.m.   Panel Discussion Among Speakers Above

5:00 p.m.   General Discussion

Day One Closing Talk

5:30 p.m.   The Vista for Developing Gene-Targeting Therapies for
             Psychiatric and Other Circuit Disorders
             STEVEN HYMAN, The Broad Institute

5:45 p.m.   Discussion

6:00 p.m.   ADJOURN DAY ONE

April 24, 2019

8:30 a.m.   Welcome and Overview of Day One
             STORY LANDIS, Co-Chair, Forum on Neuroscience and
             Nervous System Disorders (*Co-Chair*)
             LAMYA SHIHABUDDIN, Sanofi (*Co-Chair*)

SESSION III: GENE-TARGETING THERAPY TECHNOLOGIES
FOR CNS DISORDERS

Objectives:

- For different therapy modalities, and with a focus on general issues rather than specific disease indications:
  o Discuss approaches to addressing their respective administration challenges;
  o Explore CNS fluid dynamics and barriers, as well as delivery routes and distribution, and dose; and
  o Examine what is known about clinical and non-clinical safety, as well as potential long-term effects.
- Consider how previously successful approaches for spinal muscular atrophy and retinal dystrophy would need to be adapted for monogenetic disorders that have more variable onset and slower progression, and discuss timing of interventions.
- Discuss what it takes to move beyond monogenetic disorders to develop gene therapy approaches for common, heterogeneous disorders such as Alzheimer's and Parkinson's diseases.
- Examine key challenges such as:
  o CNS cell type-specific transduction;
  o Regulation of viral gene expression to optimize safety and efficacy; and
  o Capsid engineering to improve tissue-specific targeting and blood–brain barrier penetration.

8:40 a.m.   Session Overview
            DAVID BREDT, Janssen R&D (*Co-Moderator*)
            HAO WANG, Takeda Pharmaceuticals (*Co-Moderator*)

8:45 a.m.   Speakers
            BEVERLY DAVIDSON, Children's Hospital of Philadelphia and University of Pennsylvania School of Medicine
            JUNGHAE SUH, Rice University
            VIVIANA GRADINARU, California Institute of Technology
            JUDE SAMULSKI, University of North Carolina School of Medicine

9:25 a.m.   Panel Discussion

9:45 a.m.   General Discussion

10:15 a.m. BREAK

SESSION IV: CLINICAL TRIAL DESIGN
AND REGULATORY PATHWAYS

Objectives:

- **Translation and treatment paradigm:** Explore issues with pre-clinical models, delivery, considerations for first-in-human, immune response, dose–response, and dose and dose regimen selection. What unique challenges do neuropsychiatric diseases present?
- **Patient access:** Discuss recruitment challenges, natural history studies, and opportunities with registries/patient advocacy.
- **Regulatory pathway:** Address ethical considerations, issues with standards and harmonization, and overall level of proof required.
- **Risk/benefit and value to patients:** Consider how to define meaningful, clinically relevant endpoints, and how to demonstrate efficacy, safety, and overall effectiveness over the long run.
  - Specific questions may include: Should long-term toxicity studies be required (6 months or more)? Should biodistribution and rationale be considered for each gene product or can biosimilars be cross-referenced? What is a biosimilar?

10:30 a.m. Session Overview
           DANIEL BURCH, PPD Biotech (*Moderator*)

10:35 a.m. Translation
           AKSHAY VAISHNAW, Alnylam

10:45 a.m. Clinical
           MICHAEL PANZARA, Wave Biosciences
           CRISTINA SAMPAIO, CHDI Foundation

11:05 a.m. Regulatory Pathway
           PETER MARKS, Food and Drug Administration
           RUNE KJEKEN, Norwegian Medicines Agency

11:25 a.m. Ethics
           HOLLY TABOR, Stanford University

11:35 a.m. Patient Advocacy
           TIM COETZEE, National Multiple Sclerosis Society

11:45 a.m.   General Discussion

12:30 p.m.   LUNCH

SESSION V: MOVING FORWARD

Objectives:

- Discuss new technologies on the horizon, for example, non-viral approaches, small molecules targeting RNA (e.g., ExpansionRx, Arrakis, Skyhawk), chaperones, targeted protein degradation (many companies), and cell penetrant stapled peptide therapeutics (e.g., Fog Pharma).
- How can these approaches be used for psychiatric disorders and other circuit disorders?
- What else do we need to know that we do not know? Examples may include precision medicine for low-incidence disorders, developing a strategic pipeline for treatments, Timothy syndrome, and/ or neuregulins.
- Briefly discuss issues related to cost, access, and health equity, as well as AAV manufacturing capacity.

1:30 p.m.   Session Overview
FRANCES JENSEN, Perelman School of Medicine, University of Pennsylvania (*Moderator*)

1:35 p.m.   Gene Mutations in Autism and Associate Neurodevelopmental Disorders
JOSEPH BUXBAUM, Icahn School of Medicine at Mount Sinai

1:50 p.m.   Novel, Non-Viral Methods of Gene Therapy, Tunable Vectors, and AAV Manufacturing Capacity
ROBERT KOTIN, Generation Bio and University of Massachusetts Medical School

2:05 p.m.   Using a Small-Molecule Drug to Modulate Splicing
ANU BHATTACHARYYA, PTC Therapeutics

2:20 p.m.   Non-Viral Delivery Nanoplatforms for Brain-Targeted Genome Editing
SHAOQIN SARAH GONG, University of Wisconsin–Madison

2:35 p.m.   Cost, Access, and Equity Issues
             HOLLY TABOR, Stanford University

2:50 p.m.   Panel Discussion

3:05 p.m.   General Discussion

3:45 p.m.   Synthesis of Key Workshop Themes and Future Directions
             STORY LANDIS, Co-Chair, Forum on Neuroscience and
             Nervous System Disorders (*Co-Chair*)
             LAMYA SHIHABUDDIN, Sanofi (*Co-Chair*)

4:00 p.m.   ADJOURN WORKSHOP

Appendix C

Registered Attendees

Asa Abeliovich
Prevail Therapeutics

Amy Adams
National Institute of Neurological
    Disorders and Stroke

Andrew Adams
Eli Lilly and Company

Julie Adams
PPD Biotech

Diaa Ahmed
Utrecht University

Zeshan Ahmed
Eli Lilly and Company

Effie Albanis
Neurogene, Inc.

Robert Alexander
Takeda Pharmaceuticals

Reem Aljuhani
Georgetown University

Kathleen Anderson
National Institute of Mental Health

Megan Anderson Brooks
CRD Associates

Patrick Antonellis
Eli Lilly and Company

Irina Antonijevic
Wave Life Sciences

Mona Ashiya
OrbiMed

Nazem Atassi
Sanofi Genzyme

Shelli Avenevoli
National Institute of Mental Health

Jennifer Beierlein
National Science Foundation

Frank Bennett
Ionis Pharmaceuticals

Sangeeta Bhargava
National Eye Institute

Anuradha Bhattacharyya
PTC Therapeutics

Dominika Bielak
Queens College, The City University
    of New York

David Bleakman
Redpin Therapeutics

Antonello Bonci
National Institute on Drug Abuse

Carsten Bonnemann
National Institute of Neurological
    Disorders and Stroke

Lizbet Boroughs
Association of American Universities

Chris Boshoff
National Institute of Neurological
    Disorders and Stroke

Linda Brady
National Institute of Mental Health

David Bredt
Janssen R&D

Katja Brose
Chan Zuckerberg Initiative

Bob Brown
Dicerna Pharmaceuticals

Bettina Buhring
National Institute of Mental Health

Daniel Burch
PPD Biotech

Joseph Buxbaum
Icahn School of Medicine at
    Mount Sinai

Sarah Caddick
Thalamic

Rosa Canet-Aviles
Foundation for the National
    Institutes of Health

Mantej (Nimi) Chhina
BioMarin Pharmaceutical, Inc.

Lisa Chong
Science Magazine

Stephanie Ciarlone
PTC Therapeutics

Timothy Coetzee
National Multiple Sclerosis Society

Jonathan Cohen
Princeton University

Renee Corcoran
Axovant

Ronald Crystal
Weill Cornell Medicine

Bernard Dardzinski
Uniformed Services University of
   the Health Sciences

Beverly Davidson
Children's Hospital of Philadelphia
University of Pennsylvania
   Perelman School of Medicine

Paula Demassi
Ministry of Public Health of
   Uruguay

Sarah DeVos
Denali Therapeutics

Jamie Driscoll
National Institute of Mental Health

Hank Dudek
Dicerna Pharmaceuticals

Lee Dudka
Dudka & Associates

Richard Esposito
U.S. Bureau of Labor Statistics

Keith Fargo
Alzheimer's Association

Boris Feldman
Rite Aid Pharmacy

Boris Feldman
Wilson Sonsini Goodrich & Rosati

E'Lissa Flores
Milken Institute

Allyson Gage
Cohen Veterans Bioscience

Marcos Geovanini
PrevCor

Shaoqin Sarah Gong
University of Wisconsin–Madison

Joshua Gordon
National Institute of Mental Health

Viviana Gradinaru
California Institute of Technology

Julie Hagan
Apic Bio, Inc.

John Hall
IXICO

Chris Henderson
Biogen

Ross Henderson
CAREM, LLC

William Herring
Merck

Kevin Hibbert
Neurogene, Inc.

Ramona Hicks
One Mind

Mi Hillefors
National Institute of Mental Health

Richard Hodes
National Institute on Aging

Stuart Hoffman
Department of Veterans Affairs

Bruce Hope
National Institute on Drug Abuse

Nina Hsu
National Institutes of Health

Steven Hyman
The Broad Institute

Yoshimasa Ito
Eisai

Marcus Jackson
Queens College, The City University
    of New York

Anjana Jain
Food and Drug Administration

Frances Jensen
University of Pennsylvania Health
    System

Sophia Jeon
National Institute of Neurological
    Disorders and Stroke

Jeymohan Joseph
National Institute of Mental Health

Akiva Katz
University of Illinois College of
    Medicine Rockford

Petra Kaufmann
AveXis

Anastasia Khvorova
RNA Therapeutics Institute
University of Massachusetts
    Medical School

Sooja Kim
National Institutes of Health

Rune Kjeken
Norwegian Medicines Agency

Kelly Knopp
Eli Lilly and Company

Ying-Yee Kong
Department of Veterans Affairs

Jeffrey Kordower
Rush University Medical Center

Paul Korner
Axovant Gene Therapies

Walter Koroshetz
National Institute of Neurological
    Disorders and Stroke

Ana Kostic
Seaver Autism Center for Research
    & Treatment, Icahn School of
    Medicine at Mount Sinai

Robert Kotin
Generation Bio
University of Massachusetts
    Medical School

John Krystal
Yale University School of Medicine

Lina Kubli
Department of Veterans Affairs

Story Landis
National Institute of Neurological
    Disorders and Stroke

Larissa Lapteva
Food and Drug Administration

Timothy LaVaute
National Institute of Neurological
   Disorders and Stroke

Ernestine Lenteu
National Institute of Neurological
   Disorders and Stroke

Alan Leshner
American Association for the
   Advancement of Science

Liza Litvina
National Institute of Neurological
   Disorders and Stroke

Darya Litvinchuk
Apic Bio

David Litwack
Prevail Therapeutics

Laura Mamounas
National Institute of Neurological
   Disorders and Stroke

Glenn Mannheim
Food and Drug Administration

Janet Marchibroda
Bockorny Group

Peter Marks
Food and Drug Administration

Christine Marx
Duke University School of Medicine

Langston McKee
U.S. Agency for International
   Development

David McMullen
National Institutes of Health

Douglas Meinecke
National Institute of Mental Health

Fany Messanvi
National Institutes of Health

Mike Michaelides
National Institute on Drug Abuse

Enrique Michelotti
National Institute of Mental Health

Timothy Miller
PPD, Inc.

Yi Mo
Axovant Sciences

Jill Morris
National Institute of Neurological
   Disorders and Stroke

Jennifer Moser
Department of Veterans Affairs

Mattia Mroso
American Association for the
   Advancement of Science

Avindra Nath
National Institute of Neurological
   Disorders and Stroke

Rosie Stovell O'Donnell
Encoded Therapeutics

Steven Oh
Food and Drug Administration

Eileen O'Reilly
Axios

Michael Ortiz
Roivant Sciences

Maire Osborn
Dicerna Pharmaceuticals

Michael Panzara
Wave Life Sciences

Bryan Parker
International Healthcare

Tom Parry
Ovid Therapeutics

Creighton Phelps
National Institute on Aging

Keith Phillips
Eli Lilly and Company

Richard Podell
Unaffiliated

Nicole Polinski
The Michael J. Fox Foundation for
    Parkinson's Research

Jenn Poole
Takeda Pharmaceuticals

Gabriele Proetzel
Takeda Pharmaceuticals

Ronald Przygodzki
Department of Veterans Affairs

Raj Puri
Food and Drug Administration

Sesquile Ramon
Biotechnology Innovation
    Organization

Elizabeth Ramsburg
Janssen Pharmaceuticals

Kathleen Reape
Spark Therapeutics

Barbara Redman
New York University

Lorenzo Refolo
National Institute on Aging

Lauren Reoma
National Institute of Neurological
    Disorders and Stroke

Lawrence Richards
American Psychological Association

Christopher Ricupero
Columbia University Medical
    Center

Becky Roof
National Institute of Neurological
    Disorders and Stroke

Erik Runko
National Science Foundation

Cristina Sampaio
CHDI Foundation

R. Jude Samulski
University of North Carolina at
    Chapel Hill

Eric Schaeffer
Janssen R&D

Tamera Schneider
National Science Foundation

Nina Schor
National Institute of Neurological
    Disorders and Stroke

Kelly Servick
Science Magazine

Douglas Sheeley
National Institute of Dental and
    Craniofacial Research

Chun-Pyn Shen
EMD Serono, Inc.

Lamya Shihabuddin
Sanofi

John Sims
Eli Lilly and Company

Anirudh Srirangam
Roivant Sciences

Michael Steinmetz
National Eye Institute

Junghae Suh
Rice University

James Sweet
Wilson Sonsini Goodrich & Rosati

Holly Tabor
Stanford University School of
    Medicine

Edmund Talley
National Institute of Neurological
    Disorders and Stroke

Amir Tamiz
National Institute of Neurological
    Disorders and Stroke

Hiroaki Tani
Eli Lilly and Company

Anderson Umah
Neolife Health International

Akshay Vaishnaw
Alnylam

Rita Valentino
National Institute on Drug Abuse

Rosaire Verna
Georgetown University

Christina Vert
National Institute of Neurological
    Disorders and Stroke

Jeannie Visootsak
Neurogene

Bhavya Voleti
Merck

Nora Volkow
National Institute on Drug Abuse

Hao Wang
Takeda Pharmaceuticals

Shiyu Wang
Dicerna Pharmaceuticals

Jackie Ward
National Institute of Neurological
  Disorders and Stroke

Clinton Wright
National Institute of Neurological
  Disorders and Stroke

Andrew Welchman
Wellcome Trust

Rui Wu
MeiraGTx

Pamella Williams
Health Services Authority

Winifred Wu
Strategic Regulatory Partners, LLC

Doug Williamson
Lundbeck

Yining Xie
National Institutes of Health

Rachel Witten
Food and Drug Administration

Li-chiung Yang
Unaffiliated